T0123008

The Primary Care Physician's Guide to
Common Psychiatric and Neurologic Problems

The Primary Care Physician's Guide to Common Psychiatric and Neurologic Problems

Advice on Evaluation and Treatment from Johns Hopkins

EDITED BY

Phillip R. Slavney, M.D.

Eugene Meyer III Professor of Psychiatry and Medicine

AND

Orest Hurko, M.D.

Associate Professor of Neurology, Neurological Surgery, Medicine, and Pediatrics

The Johns Hopkins University School of Medicine
Baltimore, Maryland

The Johns Hopkins University Press ▪ Baltimore and London

Notice: The authors and publisher have exerted every effort to ensure that the selection and dosage of drugs discussed in this text
accord with recommendations and practice at the time of publication. The medications described do not necessarily have specific
approval by the U.S. Food and Drug Administration (FDA) for use
in the diseases and dosages for which they are recommended. The
reader should consult the package insert for each drug for use and
dosage as approved by the FDA. Because standards for usage
change, the reader should keep abreast of revised recommendations, particularly those concerning new drugs.

© 2001 The Johns Hopkins University Press
All rights reserved. Published 2001
Printed in the United States of America on acid-free paper
2   4   6   8   9   7   5   3   1

The Johns Hopkins University Press
2715 North Charles Street
Baltimore, Maryland 21218-4363
www.press.jhu.edu

Library of Congress Cataloging-in-Publication Data

The primary care physician's guide to common psychiatric and
neurologic problems : advice on evaluation and treatment from
Johns Hopkins / edited by Phillip R. Slavney and Orest Hurko.
p.   cm.
Includes bibliographical references and index.
ISBN 0-8018-6553-0 — ISBN 0-8018-6554-9 (pbk.)
1. Neurology.   2. Psychiatry.   3. Primary care (Medicine).
4. Symptoms.   I. Slavney, Phillip R. (Phillip Richard), 1940–
II. Hurko, Orest, 1948–   III. Johns Hopkins University.
RC341.P835 2001
616.8—dc21   00-010139

A catalog record for this book is available from the British Library.

For Amanda and Gordon Grender
P. R. S.

For Victoria Reed Hurko and Alexander Reed Hurko
O. H.

Contents

Contributors   ix

Preface and Acknowledgments   xi

Part I. Psychiatric Problems

1. The Screening Psychiatric Evaluation | KARIN J. NEUFELD   3
2. Sadness | JOHN R. LIPSEY   12
3. Nervousness | MICHAEL R. CLARK   35
4. Forgetfulness | PETER V. RABINS   51
5. Unrealistic Concerns about Health | MARK L. TEITELBAUM   66
6. Suicidal Thoughts | DEAN F. MACKINNON   79
7. Dependence on Alcohol or Drugs | ALAN J. ROMANOSKI   93

Part II. Neurologic Problems

8. The Screening Neurologic Evaluation | OREST HURKO   131
9. Weakness | RICHARD O'BRIEN   144
10. Numbness or Tingling | VINAY CHAUDHRY   156
11. Back Pain | JOHN DEAN RYBOCK   171
12. Headaches | DAVID W. BUCHHOLZ   179
13. Dizzy Spells | PETER W. KAPLAN   196
14. Tremor | STEPHEN G. REICH   214

Index   231

Contributors

All contributors are faculty members of the
Johns Hopkins University School of Medicine,
Baltimore, Maryland.

David W. Buchholz, M.D.
Associate Professor of Neurology

Vinay Chaudhry, M.D.
Associate Professor of Neurology

Michael R. Clark, M.D., M.P.H.
Associate Professor of Psychiatry

Orest Hurko, M.D.
Associate Professor of Neurology,
Neurological Surgery, Medicine, and Pediatrics

Peter W. Kaplan, M.B., B.S., F.R.C.P.
Associate Professor of Neurology

John R. Lipsey, M.D.
Associate Professor of Psychiatry

Dean F. MacKinnon, M.D.
Assistant Professor of Psychiatry

Karin J. Neufeld, M.D.
Assistant Professor of Psychiatry

Richard O'Brien, M.D.
Assistant Professor of Neurology

Peter V. Rabins, M.D., M.P.H.
Professor of Psychiatry

Stephen G. Reich, M.D.
Associate Professor of Neurology

Alan J. Romanoski, M.D., M.P.H.
Associate Professor of Psychiatry and Mental Hygiene

John Dean Rybock, M.D.
Assistant Professor of Neurosurgery

Mark L. Teitelbaum, M.D.
Associate Professor of Psychiatry

Preface and Acknowledgments

Primary care physicians must now evaluate and treat complaints that only several years ago were thought to need the prompt attention of specialists. These new responsibilities demand new knowledge, but many general practitioners may not have the time to read long, detailed texts; they want to understand the essence of the problem and do something to help their patients. Under the circumstances, a small book dealing with common or worrisome psychiatric and neurologic complaints should be of value to busy physicians.

Our book has 12 problem-focused chapters, the titles of which generally reflect words patients use. In each, the author describes the usual presentation of the problem in adults and enumerates its major causes. The reader is then advised on clinical assessment, initial treatment, and referral to specialists. The chapter authors define basic concepts and make practical recommendations based on their extensive experience as consultants to primary care physicians. When the first person pronoun is used, the author is giving his or her personal advice. In addition to the 12 problem-focused chapters, 2 chapters outline screening evaluations for psychiatric and neurologic disorders in general.

■ ■ ■

The editors are grateful to Wendy Harris, Joyce King, and Jacqueline Slavney for advice and assistance. Orest Hurko very much appreciates the support of SmithKline Beecham, where he was group director of Experimental Medicine in Neurosciences Discovery during the preparation of the manuscript.

PART I

Psychiatric Problems

ONE

The Screening Psychiatric Evaluation

Karin J. Neufeld, M.D.

For primary care doctors, screening for the presence of psychiatric disorders includes both reviewing specific aspects of the history and evaluating the patient's mood and cognitive ability. A skillful patient interview will facilitate early detection and appropriate treatment of psychiatric disorders, especially in patients whose initial complaints suggest nonpsychiatric illness. Although psychiatric disorders are often misunderstood and feared by the general public, an interested, matter-of-fact diagnostic approach by the primary care physician is reassuring to patients with psychiatric problems and informative to those without. Asking questions about psychiatric disorders as part of a complete medical evaluation validates their importance as common illnesses that can and should be treated.

History

Family Psychiatric History

A family history of psychiatric disorder is best elicited at the same time the rest of the family history is obtained. A positive response to a general question such as "Has anyone in your family ever had emotional problems?" should be followed with more specific questions regarding symptoms, diagnoses, and treatments. Supplementary questions such as "Has anyone in your family ever tried to harm himself or herself, or has anyone needed psychiatric treatment?" sometimes elicit important information that may go unreported with a single screening question. Knowledge that a relative has attempted or completed suicide, for example, can be very helpful to the physician in estimating the patient's risk of self-injury.

Personal Psychiatric History

Inquiries regarding the presence of psychiatric problems are most easily made within the general review of systems. Responses to questions such as "Have you ever had any emotional problems?" allow further exploration about the nature of the illness, its treatment, and the level of disability. This is especially important when the patient reports having had a "nervous breakdown," as this term has no diagnostic utility.

When patients respond in the affirmative to the initial screening question about emotional problems, the physician should ask them about thoughts of suicide. These thoughts are unlikely to be reported spontaneously by the patient and give information about the potential for self-injury. Such questions might be formulated as "Have you ever felt so bad that you wished you were dead?" or "Have you ever felt so bad that you thought of taking your life?"

Personality

Assessment of the patient's personality helps the primary care physician understand that individual's enduring strengths and weaknesses and reveals patterns of behavior that might be anticipated in times of stress. It is important to ask patients to describe themselves as they usually are, rather than how they are feeling at the moment. Information about the patient's personality obtained from other sources (e.g., family members) will aid in understanding that individual's baseline traits. Questions regarding the patient's usual mood, tendency to worry (e.g., "Are you the type of person who worries a lot, or are you relatively carefree?"), suspiciousness (e.g., "Do you tend to trust people, or do you suspect that they are taking advantage of you?"), and propensity to anger (e.g., "Are you a person who is easily angered, or does it take a great deal to get you mad?") should all be asked.

Becoming familiar with the patient's personality at baseline also allows the physician to ascertain when there has been a change from the established pattern. Such changes may indicate the onset of a psychiatric disorder. For example, the physician should consider major depression as one reason why someone who is usually cheerful and carefree has now become morose and apprehensive.

Mental Status Examination

A mental status examination should be part of any thorough clinical assessment. Some aspects of the patient's mental state can be inferred from his or her behavior, but others must be inquired about. Although family and personal psychiatric history and information about premorbid personality can be gathered adequately during the initial evaluation of the patient, the primary care physician should perform a mental status examination (however brief) at each patient encounter.

Appearance and Behavior

Observation of the patient's appearance and behavior is important to all aspects of medical examination. Many clues to underlying emotional distress or disorder can be gleaned from such observations, and the physician should note the patient's grooming, dress, degree of eye contact, facial expression, and engagement in the interaction. For example, a slumped posture, disheveled appearance, and downcast gaze may be manifestations of a major depression.

Speech and Language

It is useful to distinguish between the characteristics of speech (e.g., rate, rhythm, volume) and those of language (e.g., vocabulary, connectedness of ideas). Speech often indicates a patient's emotional state, while language reflects his or her cognitive ability. Thus, in dementia, speech may be prompt and brisk while language content is impoverished and marked by word-finding errors; in major depression, speech tends to be slow and brief, but the use of language is normal.

Mood and Suicidal Thinking

An assessment of mood is based on both the physician's observation of the patient's emotional state and the patient's responses to questions such as "What is your mood like today?" The reported mood is usually congruent with that observed; when it is not, further evaluation is needed. Most often, a mismatch occurs when someone describes feeling "OK" but appears sad and tearful. If a patient reports being sad, frustrated, or angry, it is important for the physician to ask about suicidal thoughts, as described above under "Personal Psychiatric History." Whenever the patient describes an unpleasant mood, subsequent questions (e.g., "What is upsetting you?") will flow quite naturally.

Hallucinations, Illusions, and Delusions

Hallucinations and delusions are rare among people living in the community, and their presence should lead the physician to consider disorders such as delirium, dementia, manic-depressive illness, schizophrenia, and drug abuse. Hallucinations are perceptions without stimuli and can occur in any sensory modality. Auditory and visual hallucinations are the most common types, and the physician can ask about them while reviewing the patient's hearing and vision (e.g., "Have you been hearing noises or voices that people who were with you couldn't hear?" "Have you been seeing things—with your eyes open—that people who were with you couldn't see?"). Remember that hallucinations are experienced as real perceptions, so questions such as "Did you ever hear/see/feel something that wasn't there?" may not elicit an accurate response.

Hallucinations must be distinguished from illusions, in which an environmental stimulus is misidentified (e.g., a chair is seen as a person). Illusions are more frequent in patients with sensory deficits and when stimuli are ambiguous (e.g., at dusk). Thus, although illusions can occur in psychiatric disorders, patients without such conditions also experience them.

Delusions are fixed, false, idiosyncratic beliefs. In the primary care setting, delusions of persecution, disease, and self-blame are probably the most common. Delusions may be revealed spontaneously in the course of history taking or elicited by questions such as "Have you been thinking you're ill because other people want you to suffer or are trying to hurt you?" and "Despite what I've told you, have you been worried that you have some terrible disease?" When the physician discovers hallucinations or delusions, a psychiatric consultation is almost always indicated.

Table 1.1. Median Mini-Mental State Examination Score by Age and Educational Level

| Age | Score Related to Education | | | |
	0–4 yr	5–8 yr	9–12 yr	≥12 yr
18–24	23	28	29	30
25–29	25	27	29	30
30–34	26	26	29	30
35–39	24	27	29	30
40–44	23	27	29	30
45–49	23	27	29	30
50–54	22	27	29	30
55–59	22	27	29	29
60–64	22	27	28	29
65–69	22	27	28	29
70–74	21	26	28	29
75–79	21	26	27	28
80–84	19	25	26	28
≥85	20	24	26	28

SOURCE: Adapted, with permission, from Crum et al. 1993, p. 2389. Copyright 1993, American Medical Association.

Cognitive Ability: The Mini-Mental State Examination

Cognitive impairment, which is central to delirium, dementia, and mental subnormality, often is not detected on cursory examination of an affected individual. The most widely used screening tool for assessing a patient's cognitive ability is the Mini-Mental State Examination (MMSE). The MMSE is not a diagnostic test and therefore does not indicate the cause of impairment; it is designed only to detect the presence of impairment. A perfect score is 30/30, and scores below 24 are regarded as abnormal in most individuals. As seen in Table 1.1, performance on the MMSE varies with educational level and with age. Once cognitive impairment has been detected, further history taking, psychiatric and neurologic examination, and laboratory studies are required to determine the cause of the dysfunction. The MMSE can also be used to track the course of cognitive function over time, and it is therefore helpful to obtain baseline results in individuals who are currently well but at risk for cognitive impairment.

The MMSE can be given just before the physical examination and introduced as another aspect of a thorough assessment (e.g., "I'd like to do your physical exam now, but first I'd like to test your memory, concentration, and a few other things. For example, can you tell me what the date is today?"). Instructions for using the MMSE are given in the appendix to this chapter.

REFERENCES

Crum, Rosa M.; Anthony, James C.; Bassett, Susan S.; and Folstein, Marshal F. Population-Based Norms for the Mini-Mental State Examination by Age and Educational Level. *Journal of the American Medical Association* 269 (1993): 2386–2391.

Folstein, Marshal F.; Folstein, Susan E.; and McHugh, Paul R. Mini-Mental State: A Practical Method for Grading the Cognitive State of Patients for the Clinician. *Journal of Psychiatric Research* 12 (1975): 189–198.

APPENDIX

Patient _____
Examiner _____
Date _____

"MINI-MENTAL STATE"

Maximum Score	Score	

ORIENTATION

5   ( )   What is the (year) (season) (date) (day) (month)?

5   ( )   Where are we: (state) (county) (town) (hospital) (floor).

REGISTRATION

3   ( )   Name 3 objects: 1 second to say each. Then ask the patient all 3 after you have said them. Give 1 point for each correct answer. Then repeat them until he learns all 3. Count trials and record.

Trials _____

ATTENTION AND CALCULATION

5   ( )   Serial 7's. 1 point for each correct. Stop after 5 answers. Alternatively spell "world" backwards.

RECALL

3   ( )   Ask for the 3 objects repeated above. Give 1 point for each correct.

LANGUAGE

9   ( )   Name a pencil, and watch (2 points)

Repeat the following "No ifs, ands, or buts." (1 point)

Follow a 3-stage command:

"Take a paper in your right hand, fold it in half, and put it on the floor" (3 points)

Read and obey the following:

CLOSE YOUR EYES (1 point)

Write a sentence (1 point)

Copy design (1 point)

_____ TOTAL SCORE

ASSESS level of consciousness along a continuum

Alert	Drowsy	Stupor	Coma

INSTRUCTIONS FOR ADMINISTRATION OF MINI-MENTAL STATE EXAMINATION

ORIENTATION

(1) Ask for the date. Then ask specifically for parts omitted, for example, "Can you also tell me what season it is?" One point for each correct.

(2) Ask in turn "Can you tell me the name of this hospital?" (town, county, etc.). One point for each correct.

REGISTRATION

Ask the patient if you may test his memory. Then say the names of 3 unrelated objects, clearly and slowly, about one second for each. After you have said all 3, ask him to repeat them. This first repetition determines his score (0–3) but keep saying them until he can repeat all 3, up to 6 trials. If he does not eventually learn all 3, recall cannot be meaningfully tested.

ATTENTION AND CALCULATION

Ask the patient to begin with 100 and count backwards by 7. Stop after 5 subtractions (93, 86, 79, 72, 65). Score the total number of correct answers.

If the patient cannot or will not perform this task, ask him to spell the word "world" backwards. The score is the number of letters in correct order. E.g. Dlrow = 5, dlorw = 3.

RECALL

Ask the patient if he can recall the 3 words you previously asked him to remember. Score 0–3.

LANGUAGE

Naming: Show the patient a wrist watch and ask him what it is. Repeat for a pencil. Score 0–2.

Repetition: Ask the patient to repeat the sentence after you. Allow only one trial. Score 0 or 1.

3-Stage command: Give the patient a piece of plain blank paper and repeat the command. Score 1 point for each part correctly executed.

Reading: On a blank piece of paper, print the sentence "Close your eyes" in letters large enough for the patient to see clearly. Ask him to read it and do what it says. Score 1 point only if he actually closes his eyes.

Writing: Give the patient a blank piece of paper and ask him to write a sentence for you. Do not dictate a sentence, it is to be written spontaneously. It must contain a subject and verb and be sensible. Correct grammar and punctuation are not necessary.

Copying: On a clean piece of paper, draw intersecting pentagons, each side about 1 in., and ask him to copy it exactly as it is. All 10 angles must be present and 2 must intersect to score 1 point. Tremor and rotation are ignored.

Estimate the patient's level of sensorium along a continuum, from alert on the left to coma on the right.

Source: Folstein, Folstein, and McHugh, 1975. The copyright in the Mini-Mental State Examination is wholly owned by the Mini Mental L.L.C., a Massachusetts limited liability company. For information about how to obtain permission to use or reproduce the Mini-Mental State Examination, contact John Gonsalves Jr., Administrator of the Mini Mental L.L.C., at 31 St. James Avenue, Suite 1, Boston, MA 02116, (617) 587-4215.

TWO

Sadness

John R. Lipsey, M.D.

Varieties of Sadness

Sadness is a universal human experience. Thus, patients who are sad are frequent visitors to the primary care physician's office, whether they keep their sadness a secret or express it openly.

Normal Sadness

When a sad mood is appropriate in severity and duration to the event that provoked it, is not accompanied by other psychological symptoms, and does not unduly disrupt work or social functioning, it is not pathological. We are not surprised when a fired employee, a rejected lover, or a bereaved spouse becomes sad. Such an emotional response is a natural and understandable reaction to loss. In most circumstances, it is self-limited and resolves as the patient finds new ways to adjust to adversity. In the meantime, sympathy and support may be all that is required from the physician.

Adjustment Disorder with Depressed Mood

Of course, feelings of sadness are not completely determined by circumstance. Adversity acts on individuals with particular vulnerabilities and strengths of personality that render them more or less predisposed to unhappiness. Thus, a romantic disappointment that dispirits an overly dependent person may provoke far less distress in someone more naturally self-reliant. Physicians who know their patients well will observe that a reaction of sadness depends as much on an individual's personality as on that person's circumstances. When the reaction seems inappropriately severe and persistent and evidence of a major depression is lacking, the diagnosis of an adjustment disorder with depressed mood is appropriate. Although sympathy and support from primary care physicians will help patients with this form of sadness to regain their equilibrium, formal psychotherapy is usually needed to reduce the risk of future episodes derived from the same vulnerability.

Major Depression

The varieties of sadness described above are not the most serious faced by primary care physicians in everyday practice. Sad moods may also occur as part of a psychiatric disorder in which such moods are regularly accompanied by many other morbid psychological symptoms. These symptoms unite to form a clinical state potentially devastating in its consequences. In years past, this entity was called *melancholia* or *endogenous depression;* in the most recent psychiatric nomenclature, it is called *major depression.*

It is vital that every primary care physician be skilled in the recognition of major depression because it is common, usually goes undiagnosed, causes great emotional suffering, is associated with marked social and occupational impairment, sometimes provokes suicide, and is very responsive to treatment.

Major Depression

Epidemiology

The lifetime risk of developing a major depression is 2–5 percent in men and 5–10 percent in women. Every year, 5–10 million Americans are affected. Fifty percent of those affected never seek treatment for their illness, and only half of those who do seek help have the illness appropriately diagnosed and treated.

The Syndrome of Major Depression

It is important to understand that major depression is a distinct clinical syndrome, and not simply a quantitatively more severe form of ordinary unhappiness. A sad mood is but a single symptom in the syndrome, just as cough is but a single symptom in the syndrome of pneumonia.

Major depression is characterized by (1) persistent sad or irritable mood; (2) excessive self-criticism, feelings of worthlessness, or inappropriate sense of guilt; (3) diminished mental and physical energy (abnormalities of "vital sense"); (4) insomnia or excessive sleep; (5) diminished or excessive appetite; (6) reduced sexual drive; (7) decreased capacity to experience pleasure (anhedonia); (8) wishes for death or suicidal thoughts; and (9) psychomotor retardation or agitation. Delusions and hallucinations may also occur. When they do, they tend to be congruent with the patient's mood (e.g., delusions of bodily decay, hallucinations of insulting voices).

The first three symptoms noted above (change in mood, self-attitude, and vital sense) are the central characteristics of the syndrome and are often referred to as the "depressive triad." It is common for the low mood to become increasingly unresponsive to environmental influence as the depressive episode worsens. In severe depressions, the patient becomes inconsolable and cannot be cheered by good news.

Most patients with major depression will have at least half of the symptoms listed above. As with all medical syndromes, not every patient need have every possible complaint, and the occasional patient may not experience a low mood per se (though such patients often report an absence of mood or an inability to experience pleasure). The symptoms of major depression are rarely of brief duration and should be present for at least two weeks before the physician can make the diagnosis with confidence. Untreated episodes usually last six to nine months, but may persist for a year or two.

Untreated or unsuccessfully treated major depression causes more impairment in functioning than hypertension, diabetes, arthritis, peptic ulcers, or inflammatory bowel disease. Depressed patients spend more days in bed than those with any of the above disorders, and the total economic cost of such depressions in 1990 was estimated at $44 billion in the United States. Even worse, major depression is the greatest risk factor in suicide, and 15 percent of patients with the disorder eventually kill themselves. This is made all the more tragic by the fact that such lethal outcomes can be avoided: 60 percent of depressed patients respond to the first-prescribed antidepressant, and 85 percent of all patients achieve a good outcome with appropriate therapy. These facts underline the important role primary care physicians can play in the recognition and treatment of a potentially fatal psychiatric disorder.

Bipolar Disorder

Most cases of major depression occur in patients whose episodes of illness are recurrent and relatively uniform in presentation. Each attack is similar to the last, and low mood, diminished self-esteem, and decreased energy are characteristic features. Such illnesses are diagnosed as recurrent major depression (or unipolar depression), and they can begin at any age, even in childhood. The average patient experiences four or five episodes in a lifetime, but variation from this mean is great.

A minority of patients have episodes of major depression alternating with episodes of mania. Manic illnesses are in every way the mirror image of depressive ones: the manic patient has an elated or excited mood, inflated self-esteem, heightened energy, overactivity, diminished need for sleep, racing thoughts, rapid speech, easy distractibility, and excessive interest in pleasurable activities with little regard to their consequences. Hypersexuality, excessive spending, grandiose delusions, and hallucinations (e.g., voices praising the patient) may occur. As in major depression, not every manic patient has every symptom listed above, but the triad of abnormal mood, self-attitude, and vital sense is central to the syndrome. Only about 1 percent of adults will ever experience an episode of mania, and the first attack usually occurs before age 30.

Most patients with major depression who also have episodes of elevated mood do not have frank mania. Rather, they have briefer and milder elations that are termed *hypomanias*. In these illnesses, no severe social or work-related impairment of function occurs. The patients report more rapid thinking than usual, increased energy and creativity, heightened confidence, diminished need for sleep, and a tendency to take on many projects at once. Those who know them may be amused by or may even enjoy this new state of mind if it remains relatively controlled. Delusions and hallucinations do not occur.

In the latest psychiatric classification system, patients with episodes of major depression and mania are said to have bipolar I disorder, whereas those with episodes of major depression and hypomania have bipolar II disorder.

The Etiology of Major Depression

Most cases of recurrent major depression, bipolar I disorder, and bipolar II disorder are idiopathic and probably genetic in origin. These illnesses run in families and often present generation after generation in varying degrees of severity. The concordance rate for major depression is 70 percent for identical twins and 15 percent for first-degree relatives. There appear to be multiple genetic subtypes, and inheritance seems polygenic.

Many cases of major depression are "symptomatic" rather than idiopathic; that is, they occur in the setting of clear brain pathology, endocrine disturbance, or adverse drug effects. The existence of such symptomatic cases, indistinguishable in their syndromic presentation from idiopathic major depression, gives credibility to the conceptualization of major depression as a disease of the brain.

One-quarter of patients hospitalized for acute stroke develop major depression in the weeks after their cerebrovascular accident. These poststroke depressions are more common with left frontal (cortical or subcortical) lesions, and few remit, if untreated, at six-month follow-up, even if there has been significant improvement in the neurologic deficits. Typical major depressions occur in Parkinson disease, human immunodeficiency virus (HIV) infection, and Huntington disease (in which mania can also be seen). All of these symptomatic depressions respond well to antidepressant medication.

Among the endocrine disorders that can provoke major depression are Cushing syndrome, hypothyroidism, and hyperparathyroidism. Although the mechanism for the association is not known to be endocrinologic, major depression is seen more frequently with pancreatic carcinoma than with other gastrointestinal neoplasms, and the mood disturbance often precedes local signs of the tumor.

Medications capable of inducing major depression include interferon-alpha, reserpine, methyldopa, and propranolol hydrochloride. Exogenous corticosteroids can produce states very similar to major depression and hypomania. Among abused substances, both cocaine and amphetamine withdrawal can provoke severe depressive symptoms, though these are usually of brief duration.

Diagnosing Major Depression

The diagnosis of major depression is ultimately based on clinical findings, which are obtained by a careful history and a detailed examination. The laboratory usually provides only ancillary information in the diagnostic process.

Taking a History

In general practice settings, the existence of major depression may be obscured by somatic complaints because insomnia, anorexia, diminished libido, fatigue, and feelings of ill health are common during depressive episodes. When patients have such symptoms, it is therefore important for the physician to inquire about other manifestations of a mood disorder. Moreover, medical illnesses and major depression frequently coexist, and both types of disorder deserve appropriate assessment.

Somatic Complaints and Anhedonia. In typical major depression, patients have marked insomnia, usually awakening early in the morning and not being able to fall asleep again. Sleepless hours are often distressing and filled with pessimistic or self-doubting ruminations. Sometimes, however, patients with major depression have hypersomnia: they go to bed early and arise, unrefreshed, late the next day. Because these individuals will not complain of difficulty sleeping, the physician should ask all patients who may be depressed "Has there been a change in your pattern of sleep recently?"

Changes in appetite are similarly variable. The typical patient with major depression complains of diminished appetite and consequent weight loss. Others, however, overeat (often consuming "junk" food) and gain weight with every depressive episode. The physician should therefore inquire about not only anorexia, but also *any* recent change in appetite or weight.

Questions about sexual activity are always potentially embarrassing for the patient. The most important issue is not the amount of sexual activity (which may vary with circumstance and partner), but the amount of sexual drive. A reasonably delicate approach to this topic is to say that "sometimes when people are ill they lose their interest in sex. Has that happened to you recently?" Most depressed patients, when asked in such a manner, admit to a decline in libido.

Fatigue is very common in major depression and may be one of the patient's chief complaints. Sometimes the lack of energy is so profound that patients cannot shower or dress in the morning and spend the entire day in bed, where they are listless but awake.

Many depressed patients report a lack of pleasure in daily activities. Everything seems dull and gray, and there is little enthusiasm for any undertaking. This anhedonia can be addressed by questions such as "Have you experienced a loss of pleasure in things you once enjoyed?" and "Has life been less enjoyable lately?" Another approach is to ask patients if they have recently given up any hobbies, leisure activities, or social interests. Some may admit to these changes more readily than describing a loss in the capacity for pleasure.

Precipitating Events. The occurrence of stressful life events before episodes of major depression is not uncommon early in the disorder, but as the patient gets older, episodes occur more frequently, tend to be more severe, and begin without any apparent precipitant. In fact, the presence or absence of psychosocial stressors at any age is irrelevant to the diagnosis of major depression. Moreover, situations that seem at first to have triggered a depression turn out to have been caused by it. Because depression can make people irritable, withdrawn, and inefficient, personal relationships and productivity at work eventually suffer.

Family History. The physician should always inquire about a possible family history of mood disorder, for there is a strong genetic contribution in many cases of major depression. When taking the family history, one should ask specifically about psychiatric hospitalizations and suicide.

Past Psychiatric History. Major depression is a recurrent condition in most patients, and some have experienced episodes of elated mood consistent with the diagnosis of bipolar disorder. The documentation of previous attacks should lead to the consideration of major depression as the cause of the patient's low mood, especially when current symptoms are suggestive of the disorder but not convincing.

The physician should also assess past psychiatric illnesses other than mood disorders. Panic disorder, eating disorders, and obsessive-compulsive disorder may be associated with major depression and occasionally are its earliest manifestation. Moreover, substance abuse is seen in up to a third of patients with major depression or bipolar disorder, and treatment of the mood disorder will not be successful if substance abuse persists.

Past Medical History. A medical history will undoubtedly be taken, but the physician should pay special attention to symptoms suggestive of those disorders capable of producing a symptomatic major depression.

History from Other Informants. If the patient allows it, an interview with a family member or close friend can be extremely useful. Such informants may well have observed changes in the patient that the latter is unaware of or minimizes. When depression is profound and accompanied by slowed thinking, another informant may be the only one who can give a clear history. When relatives or friends have previously seen the patient in a depressed state, they are often very aware of the initial signs of the illness. Moreover, family members may have the most accurate information about family psychiatric history.

If possible, the physician should interview other informants in the patient's presence. Separate interviews can make some patients feel belittled or even suspicious, but joint interviews tend to have a positive effect and are seldom rejected. Patients should, of course, be interviewed alone at first, so that the physician can ask them whether there are any matters they wish held in confidence at a joint meeting. Suicidal thoughts must never be kept confidential, for such secrets can have lethal results.

Examining the Patient

Mood. Although most patients reply appropriately to the question "How has your mood been recently?" some will not understand the meaning of *mood.*

When that is the case, the examiner can suggest mood terms to prompt the patient ("Have you felt low, down, or blue?") or can ask, instead, "How are your spirits?"

When patients report their mood as depressed, the physician should ask them whether it is like sadness they have experienced after disappointments or losses in the past. Many patients readily characterize the mood of major depression as both quantitatively and qualitatively distinct from that of ordinary sadness. Thus, they may say not only that their low mood is more pervasive and less responsive to external conditions, but also that it has a painful or oppressive quality absent from ordinary sadness.

The physician should also ask patients about the pattern of mood over the course of a day. Many patients describe their lowest moods in the morning, with relative or even marked improvement at night. Others experience unremitting depression during every waking hour.

Self-Attitude. Most patients with major depression have diminished self-esteem. One way for the physician to elicit such thoughts is to ask: "Sometimes when people are depressed they become very self-critical or self-doubting. I don't mean you should be having such thoughts, but I was wondering whether you are." The examiner should also ask about the patient's sense of success in his or her most prized social roles. Some patients deny diminished self-esteem on screening inquiry but later spontaneously report that they are less-capable workers, less-attractive spouses, or less-nurturing parents. Although such changes can be produced by major depression, other informants often report that the patient's ideas are distorted.

Suicidal Thinking. Whenever a patient's mood is low, the physician must inquire *directly* about wishes for death, feelings of hopelessness, and suicidal thoughts. In so doing, the examiner will decrease, rather than increase, the possibility of suicide. For advice about the assessment of suicidal thinking, see Chapters 1 and 6.

Psychomotor Abnormalities. Psychomotor retardation and agitation are signs observed during the examination. In the former, speech and movement are slow or hesitant; in the latter, rapid or impulsive. When psychomotor retardation is profound, patients can be mute and motionless.

Delusions. Delusions are common in severe cases of major depression. These fixed, false, idiosyncratic beliefs are congruent with the patient's mood. It is impossible to ask about every possible delusion, but those common in depression should be assessed. One of them, a delusional change in self-attitude, may have already been elicited. In such cases, patients may believe not only that they are worthless, harmful, or criminal individuals, but also that others (e.g., the police) are going to punish or kill them because of their transgressions. In this way, persecutory delusions occur in major depression, and patients with the disorder think the persecution is warranted.

Other depressed patients develop somatic delusions. They are not just worried about their health, as many depressed individuals are. Rather, they are convinced that they have serious and undiscovered illnesses (e.g., malignancies, AIDS). Some patients believe that they are rotting away, and no medical investigation provides reassurance. Just as frequent as somatic delusions are nihilistic ones, in which patients believe that their lives are empty and their futures bleak. When this kind of delusion is severe, depressed patients are convinced that they are alone in the world, bankrupt, or even dead.

The physician should introduce screening questions about delusions in a matter-of-fact manner that follows naturally from an understanding of the patient's mood. One such introduction is: "Sometimes when people are depressed they have distressing thoughts. I'd like to ask you about several of them." The examiner can then go on to inquire: "Have you been thinking, for example, that you're a bad person or that you deserve to suffer?" "Have you been worried that other people want to see you suffer, or even that they're trying to hurt you?" "Are you worried that you have some terrible disease—perhaps one your doctors have missed?" "Do you think you have a future?"

Hallucinations. Hallucinations are not uncommon in severe cases of major depression. Like delusions, they are congruent with mood. Auditory hallucinations are the most frequent, and patients hear voices criticizing them, berating them, telling them they are doomed, or even instructing them to commit suicide. Sensory modalities other than hearing are seldom involved. For suggestions on the assessment of hallucinations, see Chapter 1.

Using the Laboratory

Major depression is a condition that occurs in clear consciousness. If the patient's level of consciousness is altered, delirium is a far more likely diagnosis and the depressive symptoms are almost certainly secondary. The usual clinical and laboratory investigations for delirious states should be undertaken immediately, including searches for toxic, infectious, metabolic, and endocrine abnormalities, as well as structural lesions of the central nervous system (CNS). The electroencephalogram should be normal in idiopathic major depression. Urine screens for drugs of abuse are indicated if the physician suspects drug abuse but the patient denies it.

If major depression is diagnostically certain on clinical grounds, the physician should always obtain thyroid function studies. Hypothyroidism (and, more rarely, hyperthyroidism) may present with severe depression and few or no physical findings. Screening tests for other endocrine or metabolic abnormalities are usually not indicated unless the physical examination or medical history suggests them. Here, however, the physician must also consider the potential medical complications of severe depression, including dehydration, malnutrition, and the consequences of immobility (e.g., atelectasis, venous thrombosis).

Because symptomatic major depression may result from structural brain lesions, neuroimaging studies are warranted in certain circumstances. In younger, healthy patients with typical major depression and a good response to treatment, such studies are seldom fruitful. In older patients, however, unsuspected cortical and subcortical brain lesions may provoke depression or make it resistant to treatment. For this reason, neuroimaging studies are advised for patients with onset of major depression in middle age or later and for patients who are resistant to multiple trials of medication. Other indications for neuroimaging studies are atypical depressive symptoms, leading to diagnostic uncertainty, and prominent neurologic abnormalities, including cognitive impairment.

Psychiatric Referral of Depressed Patients

There are several situations in which the primary care physician should immediately refer patients with major depression to a psychiatrist. Patients with suicidal intent or a plan to kill themselves must be evaluated by a psychiatrist on an emergent basis to assess the need for psychiatric admission. If they refuse such a referral, procedures for involuntary commitment to a psychiatric hospital must be undertaken to prevent suicide, and the primary care physician should contact psychiatric colleagues for advice on how to proceed. Although uncooperative patients may be angered by such measures or may resist them, they may be grateful when they have recovered.

Patients with suicidal ideas or persistent wishes for death but no suicidal intent or plan are also best served by immediate psychiatric referral. Such patients will require frequent visits to the physician's office to make certain that they have not developed suicidal intent. Most busy general practices do not have enough flexibility to provide the intensity of care these patients deserve.

Patients who are deluded or hallucinating or who have prominent psychomotor agitation or retardation must have prompt psychiatric referral. Many will require psychiatric admission and a range of treatments beyond the reach of the generalist.

Patients at risk for malnutrition and dehydration should also be referred, but the primary care physician will be called on to manage potential medical complications as the psychiatrist speeds recovery from the depression. Patients with concurrent psychiatric illnesses (e.g., eating disorders, obsessive-compulsive disorder) should have a psychiatric consultation. Patients with a history of bipolar I disorder deserve similar referral, since antidepressant treatment can precipitate mania. Patients who have failed to respond to two antidepressant drug trials should have at least a consultation with a psychiatrist to confirm the diagnosis and to evaluate any factors hindering the response to treatment.

In any situation requiring referral to a psychiatrist, the primary care physician should make explicit the reasons for the referral so that the patient has no cause to feel rejected or abandoned. If the primary care physician has little experience or training in the treatment of mood disorders, he or she should say so plainly, for patients appreciate such honest statements. If the referral is required by severe or life-threatening symptoms or by failure to respond to initial treatments, this should also be discussed forthrightly. Secrecy regarding the reasons for referral, or surprise referral, engenders nothing but mistrust. Moreover, the chance for the patient to view the referral as an opportunity for new help, in cooperation with the primary care physician, is lost.

Finally, any patient requesting referral to a psychiatrist should be given the opportunity to have one. Such a request may simply imply that the patient is not prepared to tell the generalist the entire history. Without a history to sustain the diagnosis, few treatments in medicine can proceed effectively.

Treatment

Antidepressant drug therapy is the mainstay of treatment and is usually successful. As noted earlier, 60 percent of patients will respond to the first antidepressant used, and 85 percent respond to one of the first three agents chosen. These outcomes are possible only if medications are given in adequate doses and for an adequate length of time. Insufficient dosage and duration of therapy are the most common causes of treatment failure. Although the dosage depends on the drug, the required duration for a full therapeutic trial is six to eight weeks with most agents. Briefer trials reveal little about the true potential for drug response, and "p.r.n." use of antidepressants is useless.

This section describes the use of three classes of antidepressants—tricyclic antidepressants, selective serotonin reuptake inhibitors, and the relatively new agent venlafaxine hydrochloride—presented in the order in which they were developed. They are neither the only effective nor the most effective antidepressants. In fact, there is little evidence that any one antidepressant is superior to another, and it remains impossible to predict which patient will respond to which drug. The agents described can be most easily used by the primary care physician or have the longest "track record."

Tricyclic Antidepressants

The tricyclic antidepressants (TCAs) have been available for decades and seem to act by blocking presynaptic reuptake of norepinephrine and serotonin in the brain. These agents also cause, to varying degrees, orthostatic hypotension (due to $alpha_1$-adrenergic blockade), anticholinergic effects (secondary to antagonism of muscarinic receptors), sedation (from antihistamine action), and slowed cardiac conduction (a quinidine-like mechanism). In therapeutic doses, they do not affect cardiac output.

Despite their potential side effects, TCAs are not difficult to use if the best-tolerated agents are chosen and doses are increased gradually. Before the development of the newer antidepressants, TCAs were the treatment standard and were successfully employed—with appropriate precautions—even for elderly or medically frail persons.

Nortriptyline hydrochloride is generally the best tolerated of the TCAs, and I recommend it above other agents in the class. It has low sedative potency, has relatively mild anticholinergic effects, and causes less orthostatic hypotension than other TCAs. Another advantage is that it has a well-established "therapeutic window" of effective serum levels. These are reliably measured by many clinical laboratories and should be used to help guide treatment. A steady-state serum nortriptyline hydrochloride level between 50 and 150 ng/ml, measured 12 hours after the last dose, optimizes the chance for beneficial effect.

Before the patient begins nortriptyline hydrochloride, the physician should obtain an electrocardiogram to screen for conduction abnormalities that could be exacerbated by the drug's quinidine-like effect. The presence of such abnormalities would favor the use of a different class of antidepressants. Patients with a recent myocardial infarction, preexisting significant hypotension, bladder outlet obstruction (which might be worsened by anticholinergic effects), or a tendency to become sedated should generally not be treated with nortriptyline hydrochloride. Falls due to sedation and orthostatic hypotension are a potentially hazardous complication, especially in patients with concurrent neurologic disorders. However, with careful monitoring and gradual escalation of the dose, nortriptyline hydrochloride can often be successfully used in such cases.

Elderly patients should begin nortriptyline hydrochloride at 10 mg po qhs; if this is tolerated the first three nights, the dose is then increased to 25 mg po qhs for one week. In patients middle-aged or younger, the initial dose is 25 mg po qhs for three nights, followed by 50 mg po qhs for a week. Giving all of the medication at bedtime minimizes daytime sedation and often reduces insomnia rapidly. The low doses in the first several days help detect patients who are extremely sensitive to the sedative effects of the drug, which they may metabolize slowly.

After elderly patients have been on 25 mg po qhs for a week or younger patients on 50 mg po qhs for the same period, the physician should order a serum nortriptyline hydrochloride level to be drawn in the morning, 12 hours after the last dose. Aim for a level of 90–100 ng/ml for most patients, if they can tolerate it, and adjust the dose to attain it. Changes in dosage are made in increments of 10–25 mg per week, depending on the last serum level, the age of the patient, and tolerance of side effects. Steady-state levels are generally attained by seven days after a change in dosage.

Although most patients require 50–100 mg of nortriptyline hydrochloride per day to attain therapeutic serum levels, the occasional patient will need as little as 10 mg per day or as much as 150 mg per day. Elderly persons usually have requirements lower in this range, but variability is great in all age groups. Serum levels should be obtained about a week after dosage changes to lessen the risk of unnecessary side effects. Repeat postural blood pressure measurements are also indicated with dosage changes. Gradual dose escalation and appropriate drug-level monitoring can make tolerance of TCAs equivalent to that of the newer antidepressants. An advantage of TCAs over these latter drugs is cost: the average monthly cost of 100 mg of nortriptyline hydrochloride per day is $85.

The physician should discuss the potential side effects of TCAs with every patient before initiating treatment. Dry mouth and constipation are common but usually subside, and sedation is also possible. The physician should ask patients to contact him or her if sedation (sustained or severe) or dizziness occurs. Advise patients to arise slowly from recumbent postures, at least initially, to reduce the risk of orthostatic hypotension. Also encourage them that the side effects of TCAs generally diminish over time.

Selective Serotonin Reuptake Inhibitors

The selective serotonin reuptake inhibitors (SSRIs) are now commonly used initially in the treatment of major depression. They have a potent and selective blocking effect on the reuptake of serotonin by CNS presynaptic nerve terminals. They have weak, if any, effect on noradrenergic, dopaminergic, histaminergic, and muscarinic cholinergic receptors. Moreover, they do not have a quinidine-like effect on cardiac conduction.

The most frequently used SSRIs are fluoxetine hydrochloride, sertraline hydrochloride, and paroxetine hydrochloride, and I will discuss only these three. Because of their receptor-specific properties, these three SSRIs do not cause orthostatic hypotension, cardiac conduction abnormalities, dry mouth, constipation, or (in general) urinary retention. Sedation is relatively uncommon.

Potential side effects include nausea, anorexia, more frequent or loose stools, anxiety, restlessness, sleep disturbance (insomnia or hypersomnia), headache, diminished sexual drive, orgasmic dysfunction, and apathy. Sinus bradycardia is an uncommon side effect but is rarely symptomatic. Most of these adverse effects are mild or transient, and thus most patients tolerate SSRIs well in the short term. Over the long haul, however, up to 20 percent of patients will discontinue these drugs because of persistent changes in sexual drive or function, and a smaller number will discontinue use because of apathy, gastrointestinal disturbance, or sleep disturbance. Sertraline hydrochloride is most likely to cause diarrhea, and paroxetine hydrochloride to cause hypersomnia.

If diminished sexual drive, impotence, or anorgasmia develops during SSRI treatment, lowering the dosage of the drug may resolve the problem. If not, the physician should consider changing to a different class of antidepressant.

No strong correlation between serum levels of SSRIs and treatment outcome has been demonstrated. Thus, routine monitoring of such levels is not clinically useful.

Fluoxetine hydrochloride has a particularly long half-life: three days or more for the parent drug and a week or more for the active metabolite. For this reason, plateau levels are not rapidly achieved after changes in dosage. Paroxetine hydrochloride and sertraline hydrochloride have half-lives of about a day, similar to the TCAs.

Elderly patients can begin taking fluoxetine hydrochloride at 10 mg po qam, increasing it to 20 mg po qam after a week if the drug is well tolerated. Younger patients can usually take 20 mg po qam from the outset of treatment. Most patients begin to respond to such doses within the first several weeks. An increase to 30 mg po qam in elderly patients or 40 mg po qam in younger patients is indicated if there is no response by six weeks. Few patients require more than 40 mg per day, the average monthly cost of which is $180. If improvement is attained but intolerable side effects develop, a return to a lower dosage often solves the problem without a relapse. The patient's clinical state and fluoxetine hydrochloride's long half-life may have led to changes in dosage before plateau levels were reached, so dose reductions because of adverse effects may still keep the patient at an effective antidepressant level.

Sertraline hydrochloride is generally begun at 50 mg po qam and increased to 100 mg po qam after the first week. A subsequent increase to 150 mg po qam is made if there is no improvement by four weeks. The maximum dose is 200 mg per day, which costs approximately $180 per month.

Paroxetine hydrochloride is begun at 10 mg po qhs in elderly patients and 20 mg qhs in others. Dose increases are made to 20 or 30 mg po qhs, respectively, if there is no response in the early weeks of treatment. The maximum dose is 40 mg po qhs in elderly patients and 50 mg po qhs in younger ones. The average monthly cost of 40 mg per day is $95. Some patients find paroxetine hydrochloride sedating and tolerate it best when taken at bedtime.

The SSRIs have a wide range of potential drug interactions because of their effects on the hepatic microsomal enzyme systems. These interactions are often minor, but some can be dangerous. The metabolic inhibition of some commonly prescribed drugs by SSRIs is presented in Table 2.1.

When beginning patients on SSRIs, the physician should specifically dis-

Table 2.1. Metabolic Inhibition of Some Commonly Prescribed Drugs by Selective Serotonin Reuptake Inhibitors (SSRIs)

Drug	Metabolism Inhibited by		
	Fluoxetine hydrochloride	Sertraline hydrochloride	Paroxetine hydrochloride
Beta-blockers			
Metoprolol succinate	+	+	+
Propranolol hydrochloride	+	+	+
Timolol maleate	+	+	+
Calcium channel blockers			
Diltiazem hydrochloride	+	+	
Felodipine	+	+	
Nifedipine	+	+	
Verapamil hydrochloride	+	+	
Antiarrhythmics			
Lidocaine hydrochloride	+	+	
Quinidine gluconate	+	+	
Narcotic analgesics			
Codeine phosphate	+	+	+
Dextromethorphan hydrobromide	+	+	+
Tricyclic antidepressants			
Amitriptyline hydrochloride	+	+	+
Clomipramine hydrochloride	+	+	+
Desipramine hydrochloride	+	+	+
Imipramine hydrochloride	+	+	+
Nortriptyline hydrochloride	+	+	+
Benzodiazepines			
Alprazolam	+	+	
Diazepam	+	+	
Midazolam	+	+	
Triazolam	+	+	
Miscellaneous			
Astemizole	+	+	
Carbamazepine	+	+	
Cisapride monohydrate	+	+	
Cortisone acetate	+	+	
Cyclosporine	+	+	
Dexamethasone	+	+	
Erythromycin	+	+	
Simvastatin	+	+	
Tamoxifen citrate	+	+	

cuss the potential for sexual dysfunction. Reassure the patient that such an effect is reversible if the medication is discontinued but might also respond to a reduction in dosage. If patients are forewarned, they are far more likely to report sexual symptoms and to comply with appropriate treatment. Other side effects (e.g., nausea, sleep disturbance, anxiety) should also be discussed but have far less potential to disrupt treatment.

Venlafaxine Hydrochloride

Venlafaxine hydrochloride is chemically unrelated to the TCAs and SSRIs. At low doses, it primarily blocks the reuptake of serotonin; at moderate doses, it blocks the reuptake of both serotonin and norepinephrine. Like the SSRIs, it has no appreciable anticholinergic or antihistaminergic effects, does not block peripheral vascular alpha receptors, and does not slow cardiac conduction.

Common side effects of venlafaxine hydrochloride are nausea, dizziness, sleep disturbance, and anxiety. Of these, nausea causes the most problems, especially early in treatment. The majority of side effects are transient and relatively mild, but one is potentially serious: 5–7 percent of patients develop hypertension. This is usually mild to moderate and is related to the dose. Thus, patients treated with venlafaxine hydrochloride should have their blood pressure monitored regularly, especially when doses are increased.

Venlafaxine hydrochloride has few currently known significant drug interactions and is therefore easier to use with patients on complicated drug regimens. A potential disadvantage of venlafaxine hydrochloride is its very short half-life: 4 hours for the parent drug and 10 hours for the active metabolite. This short half-life is associated with rapid excretion of the drug if patients miss a day's doses, and some patients then develop a withdrawal syndrome manifested by dysphoria, anxiety, dizziness, and complaints of peripheral "electrical" sensations. The withdrawal syndrome may occur even with the sustained-release formulation.

Venlafaxine hydrochloride is usually begun as the immediate-release formulation, 37.5 mg po bid taken with meals to reduce nausea. Elderly patients or those sensitive to nausea may need to start at 18.75 mg po bid. I then slowly increase the dose to 75 mg po bid by the end of the second or third week. Few patients, in my experience, respond to lower doses. If the total dose of 150 mg per day is ineffective after four or five weeks, an increase to 225 mg per day in divided doses is warranted. Immediate-release venlafaxine hydrochloride must always be given on at least a twice daily schedule because of its rapid excretion. Occasional patients require up to

375 mg per day. The average monthly cost of 225 mg of immediate-release venlafaxine hydrochloride per day is $150.

Sustained-release venlafaxine hydrochloride may be given once a day, at mealtime. Dosage begins at 37.5 mg po qd for several days and then increases to 75 mg po qd, with a goal of 150 mg po qd by two or three weeks. If there is no response to treatment by the fourth or fifth week, an increase to 225 mg po qd is indicated. The manufacturer does not as yet recommend doses of more than 225 mg of this formulation per day.

In addition to discussing common side effects and the potential for hypertension, the physician should warn all patients about uncomfortable withdrawal reactions if they suddenly discontinue the drug. Whenever possible, venlafaxine hydrochloride should be tapered over several weeks before it is stopped.

Choosing an Antidepressant

Which antidepressant—nortriptyline hydrochloride, an SSRI, or venlafaxine hydrochloride—should be started first? There is, really, little difference among them in terms of treatment efficacy. Rather, potential side effects, the individual patient's acceptance of those side effects, and comorbid medical conditions should determine which agent to use first. For instance, nortriptyline hydrochloride would not be a good choice for a patient with poorly controlled orthostatic hypotension but might be excellent for a medically stable patient with severe insomnia. An SSRI might be ideal for a patient with severe constipation, but someone unwilling to accept any adverse effect on sexual function would tolerate it poorly. Similarly, venlafaxine hydrochloride might be easier to give to patients on several other medications but would predictably lead to withdrawal symptoms in those prone to skip drug doses.

After the physician chooses the first antidepressant agent, the transition to the next class sometimes requires caution. In particular, changes from nortriptyline hydrochloride to an SSRI, or the reverse, have the potential for SSRI-induced inhibition of nortriptyline hydrochloride excretion. This usually causes little difficulty if nortriptyline hydrochloride is tapered over several days and an SSRI is then slowly introduced. However, SSRI-induced inhibition of P450IID6 hepatic microenzymes may lead to substantially elevated and potentially toxic levels of nortriptyline hydrochloride if nortriptyline is begun and the dose increased in close proximity to an SSRI. This is particularly so for fluoxetine hydrochloride, as its prolonged half-life may sustain therapeutic levels of the drug for *weeks* after its discontinuation. In this situation, nortriptyline hydrochloride doses must be very low at first, and serum nortriptyline levels must be monitored regularly. Conversely, once fluoxetine hydrochloride is fully cleared, nortriptyline hydrochloride doses that were initially adequate to attain therapeutic serum levels may have to be increased.

Explaining Major Depression and Its Treatment

Whichever antidepressant is chosen, the physician must always reassure patients of his or her assessment of the illness and the prospects for recovery. Tell patients, in a straightforward manner, that major depression is a medical condition; it is not, in *any* sense, a character flaw or a weakness of personality. Antidepressant agents are medical treatments, not psychological crutches. Although patients are responsible for cooperation in their treatment and for reasonable behavior during their recovery, they are by no means responsible for their psychiatric illness.

Discuss prognosis in openly optimistic terms because the great majority of patients with major depression recover with appropriate treatment. Recurrences can often be prevented or diminished in intensity or frequency. Such a prognosis is certainly better than that of most chronic medical conditions, and depressed patients are reassured to hear it. Until recovery occurs, reassurances are well worth repeating.

Carefully explain to patients the time course of recovery with antidepressants. Patients who are informed about the necessity for full treatment trials, the possible six- to eight-week response time, and the need to switch antidepressant should one fail are far more likely to maintain hope than patients who expect that recovery will occur overnight.

Finally, the physician can advise recovered patients that maintenance antidepressant treatment is often indicated. The great majority of patients who have experienced one major depression will have recurrences. The frequency of such recurrences is greatly diminished by prophylactic treatment. If a patient has had only one episode, a case can be made for slow tapering of the antidepressant after a year of treatment, with careful monitoring for relapse. After a second episode, the physician may advise patients to remain on antidepressants indefinitely.

Summary

Major depression is a common, often severe, and potentially life-threatening syndrome. Typical features include persistent sadness, excessive self-doubt, diminished mental and physical energy, disturbed sleep and appetite, decreased capacity to experience pleasure, and wishes for death or suicidal ideas. Major depression is not simply a more severe form of ordinary unhappiness. Only 50 percent of patients with major depression ever seek treatment for their illness, and only half of those who do are appropriately diagnosed and treated. In many cases, the first opportunity to detect the illness occurs in primary care settings. The diagnosis of major depression should not be made without a thorough examination of the patient's mental state and a careful review of his or her past psychiatric history. Information obtained from members of the patient's family can be crucial for accurate diagnosis. Uncomplicated cases of major depression can be treated by primary care physicians. Treatment with antidepressants is effective in more than 80 percent of patients. Patients whose illnesses do not respond to a course of antidepressant medication, patients who have additional psychiatric disorders, and patients who are profoundly depressed, delusional, or suicidal are best served by referral to a psychiatrist.

REFERENCES

Coyne, James C.; Schwenk, Thomas L.; and Fechner-Bates, Suzanne. Nondetection of Depression by Primary Care Physicians Reconsidered. *General Hospital Psychiatry* 17 (1995): 3–12.

Greenberg, Paul E.; Stiglin, Laura E.; Finkelstein, Stan N.; and Berndt, Ernst R. The Economic Burden of Depression in 1990. *Journal of Clinical Psychiatry* 54 (1993): 405–418.

Hyman, Steven E.; Arana, George W.; and Rosenbaum, Jerrold F. *Handbook of Psychiatric Drug Therapy,* 3d ed., pp. 43–92. Boston: Little, Brown, 1995.

Olfson, Mark; Fireman, Bruce; Weissman, Myrna M.; Leon, Andrew C.; Sheehan, David V.; Kathol, Roger G.; Hoven, Christina; and Farber, Leslie. Mental Disorders and Disability among Patients in a Primary Care Group Practice. *American Journal of Psychiatry* 154 (1997): 1734–1740.

Schulberg, Herbert C.; Block, Marian R.; Madonia, Michael J.; Scott, C. Paul; Rodriguez, Eric; Imber, Stanley D.; Perel, James; Lave, Judith; Houck, Patricia R.; and Coulehan, John L. Treating Major Depression in Primary Care Practice: Eight-Month Clinical Outcomes. *Archives of General Psychiatry* 53 (1996): 913–919.

Wells, Kenneth B.; Stewart, Anita; Hays, Ron D.; Burnam, M. Audrey; Rogers, William; Daniels, Marcia; Berry, Sandra; Greenfield, Sheldon; and Ware, John. The Functioning and Well-being of Depressed Patients: Results from the Medical Outcomes Study. *Journal of the American Medical Association* 262 (1989): 914–919.

THREE

Nervousness

Michael R. Clark, M.D., M.P.H.

The word *nervous* means unnaturally or acutely uneasy or apprehensive. In many situations a sense of nervousness or anxiety is appropriate. Normal anxiety serves as an alerting signal of impending danger, enables the person to prepare for and deal with stress, and is clearly adaptive in problem solving and being productive. Anxiety affects levels of arousal, cognitive functions such as attention and concentration, and physiologic systems such as the cardiovascular and gastrointestinal. Many patients are appropriately anxious about symptoms, diagnoses, tests, treatments, and prognoses of their medical problems. Information and reassurance will usually calm them. However, a significant number of patients experience pathological anxiety that interferes with their functioning and may explain their somatic complaints.

Inappropriate and sustained stress-response mechanisms are probably a component of pathological anxiety states. Pathological anxiety can take several forms but is usually experienced as a sense of apprehension without obvious danger or fear in a situation that most people would not find threatening. The psychological and physiologic dysfunction of patients with anxiety disorders is comparable to that of patients with chronic medical illnesses such as diabetes mellitus and congestive heart failure, and the majority of them seek professional help and take medications. Primary care physicians have an excellent opportunity to recognize anxiety disorders and initiate treatment or referral, with resulting resolution of patients' distress and return to premorbid levels of function.

Epidemiology

Anxiety disorders are the most common psychiatric illnesses in both the general population and the general medical setting. The lifetime prevalence of anxiety disorders has been estimated at 25 percent, and up to a third of patients in primary care meet screening criteria for such conditions. The usual onset of anxiety disorders is in early adulthood, and they occur more often in women than in men. Table 3.1 summarizes the distinguishing features of four common anxiety disorders: generalized anxiety disorder, panic disorder, obsessive-compulsive disorder, and social phobia.*

Patients with anxiety disorders are more likely to complain of somatic symptoms than psychological ones. In a study of five hundred anxious or depressed primary care patients, 84 percent presented with somatic complaints, while only 17 percent presented with psychological symptoms. When psychological symptoms were described, the correct diagnosis was made 94 percent of the time; when somatic complaints were described, the correct diagnosis was made only 50 percent of the time. Another study found that the prevalence of anxiety disorders was 31–35 percent in patients complaining of abdominal pain, chest pain, or insomnia.

There is also a strong positive correlation between the number of physical complaints patients experience and the likelihood that they have an anxiety disorder. For example, fewer than 10 percent of patients with two or three somatic complaints were found to have an anxiety disorder, as compared to 48 percent of patients with more than eight somatic complaints. Such findings emphasize the importance of assessing psychological symptoms, regardless of a patient's chief or presenting complaint.

Patients with anxiety disorders are high utilizers of medical services and have much greater health-care costs than other patients, even after adjustment for concurrent medical conditions. This effect is evident in a study of one large health maintenance organization (HMO), in which the top 10 per-

---

* Patients with chronic anxiety about their health (hypochondriasis) are discussed in Chapter 5. Patients with anxiety after severe physical or emotional trauma (posttraumatic stress disorder) often have "flashbacks" and nightmares and should be referred to a psychiatrist for treatment.

Table 3.1. Distinguishing Features of Common Anxiety Disorders

Feature	Generalized Anxiety Disorder	Panic Disorder	Obsessive-Compulsive Disorder	Social Phobia
Type of anxiety	Sustained vague worry	Overpowering dread	Specific but excessive worry	Fear of embarrassment
Onset	Gradual	Sudden	Gradual	Sudden
Precipitant	No	Rare	No	Yes
Situational	No	Sometimes	Sometimes	Yes
Autonomic symptoms	±	++	−	+
Associated behavior	Gradual restrictions in usual daily activities	Avoidance of situations associated with attacks	Time-consuming repetitive or stereotyped rituals	Avoidance of specific situations
Course	Chronic	Episodic	Chronic	Episodic

cent of health-care utilizers were compared to the bottom 50 percent. The top 10 percent had more primary care visits (29% vs. 18%), outpatient specialty visits (52% vs. 7%), and hospital days (48% vs. 9%). In this top 10 percent, persistent anxiety was one of the most common causes that led patients to see physicians.

Usual Presentations of Common Anxiety Disorders

Subsyndromal Anxiety

In the primary care setting, patients sometimes complain of anxiety symptoms that do not meet diagnostic criteria for an anxiety disorder. These patients usually report brief or intermittent anxiety in the setting of stresses such as bereavement, serious illness, marital discord, or financial embarrassment. The patients are often anxiety-prone individuals and describe themselves as worriers at baseline. Treatment of subsyndromal anxiety includes emotional support and medications to control symptoms (see below).

Generalized Anxiety Disorder

Generalized anxiety disorder (GAD) is characterized by excessive and uncontrollable worry lasting weeks or months, with restlessness, fatigue, muscular tension, poor concentration, irritability, and insomnia. Patients usually deny symptoms of autonomic hyperactivity. The patient's worry is not focused on a single issue (e.g., health) but invades all aspects of daily life, even when other informants report that the patient has few causes for concern.

Approximately two-thirds of patients with GAD have a concurrent psychiatric disorder, and over 90 percent of patients with a lifetime diagnosis of GAD have at least one other lifetime psychiatric diagnosis. The most common comorbid illnesses include phobias, panic disorder, and depressive disorders. Controversy exists as to whether GAD is an independent entity, a prodrome to another disorder, or a residual form of a previous illness.

Regardless of the actual nature of GAD, patients who have the condition report a five-year duration of symptoms on average and significant interference with their daily activities. A third receive some type of public assistance, and only half work full-time. As with all severe anxiety disorders, patients have a high probability of seeking professional help and of using medications to control symptoms.

Panic Disorder

In contrast to GAD, panic disorder is characterized by attacks of sudden, intense fear or discomfort associated with various combinations of shortness of breath, palpitations, chest pain, sweating, trembling, nausea, dizziness, paresthesias, restlessness, chills, hot flashes, depersonalization, and a sense of losing control or impending death. These episodes usually occur without warning and reach a peak within 10 minutes. When symptoms are severe, many patients believe they are having a myocardial infarction and call an ambulance. Although panic attacks last less than an hour, they can leave a person feeling ill for several hours or even days afterward. Once patients have had a few attacks, they become preoccupied with the possibility of having another.

Patients with panic disorder may or may not have agoraphobia. This latter condition is defined as fear of situations in which help might not be available. As a result of agoraphobia, individuals with panic disorder may become housebound or leave their homes only in the company of another person. Agoraphobia without a history of panic disorder is rare.

A third of patients with panic disorder have a concurrent major depression, and two-thirds have a lifetime risk of that disorder. Some patients with panic disorder abuse alcohol in an attempt to diminish their symptoms, while others inadvertently provoke attacks by using cocaine or amphetamines.

Forty-three percent of patients with panic disorder are first seen in an emergency department, and 35 percent are first seen in a primary care setting. If such patients complain primarily of somatic symptoms rather than anxiety or depression, an accurate diagnosis is made only half the time. As a result, patients with panic disorder have usually seen more than 10 physicians and have sought evaluation for more than a decade before their illness is correctly identified.

Although patients with panic disorder have increased rates of peptic ulcer disease and hypertension, as well as a mildly elevated risk for death from cardiovascular causes, they commonly report somatic symptoms for which no cause other than panic disorder can be found. Cardiopulmonary, gastrointestinal, and neurologic complaints are especially frequent. Only 10 percent of patients present with psychological symptoms or describe their somatic complaints as psychological in origin. Patients of cardiologists and gastroenterologists have rates of panic disorder ranging from 29 percent to 98 percent, depending on the type of investigation involved.

Obsessive-Compulsive Disorder

Obsessive-compulsive disorder (OCD) is found in 1–2 percent of the general population. Patients experience recurrent thoughts (obsessions) accompanied by anxiety. The obsessions are often followed by repetitive behavioral or mental acts (compulsions) to prevent or reduce that anxiety. Thus, patients with obsessional doubts about having locked a door or ridding their hands of germs will repeatedly check the lock or scrub their hands to the point of severe dryness and cracking of the skin.

In primary care settings, patients with OCD may report feeling anxious or depressed, but many will not spontaneously describe their obsessions and compulsions for fear of being thought "crazy" by their physician. For this reason, the primary care physician should ask all anxious patients about obsessions and compulsions. For example, when trying to elicit obsessions, I ask: "Sometimes people have repetitive or even silly thoughts that intrude into their minds. Do you ever have thoughts like that?" If I want to discuss compulsive behaviors, I might say: "Similarly, people can feel the need to perform certain acts over and over again, such as washing their hands or touching an object a particular number of times. Do you ever do things like that?"

Social Phobia

Social phobia is defined as a marked or persistent fear of social or performance situations in which an individual is exposed to unfamiliar people or to possible scrutiny by others. Patients with social phobias are apprehensive about acting in a fashion that will be humiliating or embarrassing. When the situation cannot be avoided, anxiety is provoked and may reach the severity of a panic attack.

Physicians underrecognize social phobias despite the fact that these are sometimes associated with significant impairment and abuse of alcohol and other sedatives. In general, patients with social phobias are twice as likely to be prescribed psychotropic medications (especially benzodiazepines) as are other patients in primary care.

Clinical Assessment

Excluding Medical Disorders That Can Mimic Anxiety Disorders

Just as anxiety disorders can mimic or complicate medical disorders, medical disorders can mimic or complicate anxiety disorders. Patients who complain of persistent or intermittent nervousness, with or without somatic symptoms, should therefore be evaluated for conditions such as hyperthyroidism, hypoglycemia, anemia, hypoparathyroidism, cardiac arrhythmias, and pheochromocytoma.

After a thorough history and physical examination that will rule out most medical disorders, the primary care physician should order a complete blood count (CBC), chemistry panel, thyroid function tests (TFTs), and an electrocardiogram (ECG). Other investigations (e.g., urinary or plasma catecholamines) should be performed when specific conditions (e.g., pheochromocytoma) are suspected. Although mitral valve prolapse is sometimes found on echocardiogram in patients with panic disorder, the relationship is almost certainly coincidental.

Screening for Anxiety Disorders and Psychosocial Problems

When patients report both anxiety and somatic complaints, it is easy to assume that their apprehensiveness is a result of their medical condition. That is often true, of course, but sometimes the opposite relationship holds. Even when a medical disorder is present, not all anxiety is "normal." Anxiety disorders are significantly more common in patients with chronic medical illnesses than in those without. Furthermore, anxiety disorders can provoke, maintain, or worsen certain medical conditions (e.g., hypertension, gastroesophageal reflux, myofascial pain). Whether or not a patient has a medical disorder, then, nervousness or worry should prompt a search for an anxiety disorder.

Screening for psychiatric disorders is important in the evaluation of any patient, and specific methods exist for the detection of anxiety disorders in the primary care setting. The use of such questionnaires and brief interviews during routine office visits improves the recognition of psychiatric disorders and reduces the stigma associated with emotional complaints.

The PRIME-MD is one of several screening tools for psychiatric disorders in primary care settings. The patient completes a brief questionnaire, which includes three items about experiencing anxiety attacks, feeling on edge, and worrying a lot. For anxiety disorders, the questionnaire's sensitivity is 94 percent and specificity is 53 percent. If any of the items is answered in the affirmative, the clinician evaluates the patient with specific questions designed to elicit the diagnostic criteria of GAD, panic disorder, and anxiety disorder not otherwise specified. For the clinician evaluation, sensitivity is 69 percent and specificity is 90 percent. Approximately eight minutes is required for a primary care physician to complete this evaluation.

The "BATHE" approach is useful in screening for psychosocial problems. The first component of the assessment is *background* information and begins with the question "What is going on in your life?" The goal of this inquiry is to elicit specific descriptions rather than the general, conventional responses that tend to follow the question "How are you doing?" The patient's *affect* is next assessed by asking "How do you feel about that?" This question emphasizes that emotional responses to situations or symptoms are clinically important.

The physician or nurse then asks "What is it about the situation that *troubles* you the most?" The answer is likely to reveal why the patient has actually come for help. Once this information is obtained, the goals of treatment from the patient's point of view are clarified. The next step is to learn how the patient is coping by asking "How are you *handling* that?" Here, the emphasis is not only on specific attempts to solve the problem, but also on how the patient's functioning has been affected by it.

This brief psychosocial assessment ends with an expression of *empathy* by the physician or nurse. Patients need to be reassured that their problems will be taken seriously. A general statement (e.g., "That must be very difficult") acknowledges the patient's complaints and communicates an understanding of the situation. The physician can then offer more specific support and make a transition to further evaluation or initial treatment.

The Treatment of Anxiety Disorders in Primary Care

Once the primary care physician has made the diagnosis of an anxiety disorder, treatment can begin. The first step is not to prescribe a medication or refer the patient to a psychiatrist or psychologist, but to reinforce the doctor-patient relationship. The physician should review the key elements that went into making the diagnosis; this review will clarify the fact that an anxiety disorder is not a diagnosis of exclusion or of last resort, made only because the physician has no other explanation for the patient's complaints. Next, the physician should educate the patient about the existence of effective treatments, including medications, psychotherapy, and behavior therapy. Finally, the physician should outline an initial treatment plan. This will reassure patients that their physician will not abandon them, will continue to direct their medical care, and will request input from specialists when needed.

Generalized Anxiety Disorder

The optimal treatment plan for GAD includes medication. The three types of medication most commonly prescribed are azapirones, benzodiazepines, and antidepressants. The selection of a particular type will depend on the nature and severity of the patient's symptoms and on the side effects of the chosen drug. Although benzodiazepines are often prescribed for GAD and can produce short-term benefit, they are not recommended for long-term treatment because they induce physiologic dependence. Patients with less severe GAD should be started on buspirone hydrochloride, while those with more severe GAD will probably require an antidepressant to control their symptoms.

The azapirone buspirone hydrochloride is a weak antagonist of 5-HT$_{1A}$ receptors and has few side effects. The initial dose is 5 mg po tid, and the medication can be titrated up to 20 mg tid if needed. (The monthly cost of the drug at this latter dose is about $260.) Buspirone hydrochloride is unlikely to interact with other medications or alcohol, to disinhibit patients, or to cause cognitive impairment or delirium. In addition, since buspirone hydrochloride causes no euphoria or physiologic dependence, there is little potential for abuse and no withdrawal syndrome if it is stopped abruptly. Buspirone hydrochloride takes one to three weeks to act, unlike benzodiazepines, which can produce relief of anxiety within minutes.

Antidepressants that block reuptake of biogenic amines (serotonin, norepinephrine, dopamine) generally require longer periods of treatment to demonstrate efficacy in anxiety disorders than do buspirone hydrochloride or benzodiazepines. If patients have accompanying symptoms of depression, they are more likely to be helped by antidepressant medications. Maintenance treatment with antidepressants is generally associated with low risks. Side effects usually occur early in treatment, before the drug's benefits are realized.

Although the anxiolytic properties of antidepressants were first observed with tricyclic antidepressants (TCAs) and monoamine oxidase inhibitors, the selective serotonin reuptake inhibitors (SSRIs) are now preferred because they are safer and usually well tolerated. In general, dosing should start with the lowest possible amount once a day (e.g., paroxetine hydrochloride, 10 mg po qhs; sertraline hydrochloride, 25 mg po qam). The dose should be increased until symptoms remit or intolerable side effects occur. Therapeutic doses are usually similar to those used to treat major depression (e.g., paroxetine hydrochloride, 40 mg po qhs; sertraline hydrochloride, 200 mg po qam), but some patients may need higher doses. The approximate monthly cost of paroxetine hydrochloride, 40 mg per day, is $160; that for sertraline hydrochloride, 200 mg per day, is also $160.

Case Example: A 52-year-old woman complained to her primary care physician of insomnia, muscle tension, and fatigue. Her general health had been good, save for mild osteoarthritis and well-controlled hypertension. She had had an episode of severe depression after the birth of her second child but had not sought treatment and her mood had gradually returned to normal after about a year.

On questioning by her physician, she described a sense of worry about family members becoming ill or having an accident. She realized these concerns were excessive, but she was nonetheless preoccupied with them for most of the day. Of late, she had been having trouble keeping up with her housework and had stopped socializing with her close friends. Although her worrying had been present on and off for years, it was becoming more intense and persistent.

A previous physician had once treated her with diazepam, 5 mg po bid, with an occasional extra dose at bedtime when she had difficulty going to sleep. She had felt much better with the medication and had stopped it on her own after a few months, without recurrence of anxiety or development of withdrawal.

The patient's physical examination was normal, save for a slightly elevated systolic blood pressure, degenerative changes in several joints, and mild obesity. CBC, chemistry panel, TFTs, ECG, and chest x-ray were normal.

The diagnoses of GAD and probable past major depression were made, and sertraline hydrochloride, 25 mg qam, was prescribed. Two weeks later the patient felt better but was still apprehensive. The dose of sertraline hydrochloride was gradually increased to 100 mg qam, and a month later the patient reported that she had not felt so well in years. She had resumed all of her usual activities and decided to take an art class at the local community college.

Panic Disorder

The role of medications, especially antidepressants, in the treatment of panic disorder is well established. Both TCAs and SSRIs have been used successfully, with over two-thirds of patients reporting remission of symptoms after 12 weeks of treatment. If a TCA is selected, nortriptyline hydrochloride or desipramine hydrochloride should be used because these have fewer side effects than other medications in their class. Initial doses are 10 mg po qhs for nortriptyline hydrochloride and 25 mg po qhs for desipramine hydrochloride. Serum drug levels should be monitored as doses are increased to maintenance ranges of 50–100 mg qhs for nortriptyline hydrochloride and 100–200 mg qhs for desipramine hydrochloride. The approximate monthly cost for nortriptyline hydrochloride, 100 mg qhs, is $50; for desipramine hydrochloride, 200 mg qhs, it is $40. The SSRIs do not require monitoring of serum levels, but they can cause significant drug-drug interactions (see Table 2.1). Maintenance doses of SSRIs for panic disorder are similar to those used for GAD, though patients with panic disorder can often tolerate higher initial doses (e.g., paroxetine hydrochloride, 20 mg qhs; sertraline hydrochloride, 50 mg qam).

Although benzodiazepines have significant side effects, they are potent anxiolytics with a rapid onset of action and a wide margin of safety. Patients with frequent or intense panic attacks are likely to require a benzodiazepine initially, especially if they experience prominent adrenergic symptoms. Lorazepam is a most useful drug in this class because of its short to intermediate half-life (approximately 12 hours), lack of active metabolites, relative safety in the presence of liver disease, and preparation in both oral and parenteral forms. A typical starting dose of lorazepam in panic disorder is 0.5 mg po tid, with maintenance doses of 1 mg po tid (approximate monthly cost, $52). Geriatric patients may tolerate oxazepam better than lorazepam because its more gradual onset of action is less likely to produce cognitive side effects. A typical starting dose for oxazepam is 10 mg po tid.

Benzodiazepines with short or very short half-lives (e.g., alprazolam, zolpidem tartrate) should be avoided because of the high potential for abuse and the high rate of withdrawal symptoms on discontinuation. Long-acting agents are preferable to very-short-acting ones to stabilize a patient's condition because they minimize these risks. One such long-acting benzodiazepine is clonazepam, which can be prescribed in an initial dose of 0.5 mg po bid. All benzodiazepines are capable of inducing memory loss that does not diminish with duration of treatment.

The short-term benefits of benzodiazepines must be balanced against the likelihood that long-term treatment will be needed. Long-term treatment increases the risk of rebound anxiety or withdrawal after the drug is stopped. Most often, patients with panic disorder will require a benzodiazepine for one to two months to control their attacks until an antidepressant regimen is established. In this situation, after the maintenance dose of the antidepressant is reached, the benzodiazepine is gradually tapered and discontinued over three to six weeks.

Case Example: A 45-year-old man with an increasingly stressful job, well-controlled hypertension, and a history of recurrent peptic ulcers presented to his primary care physician after going to an emergency room the night before with chest pain, shortness of breath, nausea, dizziness, and fear that he was having a heart attack. In the emergency room his blood pressure was 180/100 and his pulse 110. An ECG showed sinus tachycardia and nonspecific ST segment changes, but no signs of ischemia or conduction abnormality. The patient insisted that blood tests be performed, and all studies were normal, including creatine kinase MB isoenzyme level.

In his physician's office, the patient was apprehensive because he was certain that pressures at work had finally caught up with him and that a serious illness was present. He reluctantly admitted having had similar attacks with increasing frequency over the past six months. He had ignored these attacks, hoping that they were indigestion, muscle strain, or "just stress."

The patient asked to have a cardiac catheterization and gastrointestinal endoscopy to evaluate the cause of his pain. His physician suggested a treadmill stress test instead and explained that the clinical picture was characteristic of panic disorder. The physician said that he would like to start the patient on medication and assess his response. He prescribed clonazepam, 0.5 mg bid, and asked the patient to stop drinking alcohol.

A week later the patient reported that he had had only one attack and that it was much less severe than previous ones. With that history, the physician concluded that the diagnosis of panic disorder was virtually confirmed and that the patient should be treated with prophylactic medication. Under the circumstances, the patient agreed to postpone the stress test. His physician prescribed paroxetine hydrochloride, 20 mg po qhs, and continued the clonazepam for a month. On follow-up, the patient reported only one mild attack and agreed to taper and discontinue the clonazepam over the next two weeks. He then continued on paroxetine hydrochloride without panic attacks or side effects, and the stress test was canceled.

Other Anxiety Disorders

Because patients with OCD usually require high doses of SSRIs and because cognitive and behavioral therapies are important in the treatment of OCD and social phobias, the primary care physician should refer patients with these disorders to a psychiatrist once the diagnosis is entertained.

Referral to Mental Health Professionals

Several types of mental health professionals are available, including psychiatrists, psychologists, social workers, and nurse therapists. The nature of the clinical problem should determine which of these is most appropriate to treat an anxious patient. For example, prompt referral to a psychiatrist is indicated if the patient has severe symptoms that impair daily functioning or are associated with suicidal thoughts. A psychiatrist should also be selected when there is diagnostic uncertainty; when advice is needed about medications; when the patient has complicated medical comorbidity; when another psychiatric condition, such as major depression, substance abuse, or personality disorder, is present; and when the anxiety is due to OCD or posttraumatic stress disorder. In addition, psychiatrists should be able to design pharmacologic treatments for patients whose disorder has failed to respond completely to initial medication trials by primary care physicians.

Psychological treatments are important for patients with anxiety disorders. Psychologists, social workers, and nurse therapists specialize in psychological treatments, and primary care physicians should consult them when referral to a psychiatrist is not required or preferred. Psychiatrists themselves refer patients to other mental health professionals for cognitive-behavioral therapies and when the psychiatrists wish to focus on the pharmacologic aspects of treatment.

Psychotherapy incorporating cognitive-behavioral techniques is usually performed by psychologists. Among such techniques are cognitive restructuring (e.g., formulating alternatives to anxious thoughts), relaxation training and biofeedback, and systematic desensitization to anxiety-provoking stimuli. Social workers and nurse therapists are more likely to specialize in psychotherapy focusing on issues such as conflicts in the patient's life, difficulties in relationships, and feelings of loss and demoralization.

The Prognosis of Anxiety Disorders

Although most patients with anxiety disorders improve with treatment, many need long-term follow-up. The primary care physician should decrease or discontinue medications after patients have been asymptomatic for six months but should vigorously reinstitute treatment at the first sign of relapse.

Patients with GAD have been found to be symptomatic for 56 percent of their lives after the onset of symptoms. The risk of relapse in GAD is high: up to 25 percent in the first month after discontinuation of treatment; up to 80 percent in the first year. Because patients treated for longer than six months have a lower rate of relapse, this should be the minimal duration of therapy before the physician attempts to decrease the dose of medication. Recent studies have found that integrated treatment combining pharmacotherapy and cognitive-behavioral techniques produces longer periods of remission after the discontinuation of drugs.

Patients with panic disorder have been found to be symptomatic for 16 percent of their lives after the onset of their illness. For panic disorder with agoraphobia, the figure is 29 percent. Despite this relatively good prognosis, the relapse rate in panic disorder is 80 percent within two years after stopping treatment, and up to 20 percent of patients are chronically ill. Patients with agoraphobia, major depression, substance abuse, or personality disorders have poorer treatment outcomes, as do those who discontinue their medications without their physician's advice. Rates of suicide attempts by patients with panic disorder have been as high as 20 percent.

Improvement rates in untreated OCD have varied from 32 percent to 74 percent. The longest prospective study examined patients an average of 47 years after a psychiatric inpatient admission. Although over 80 percent of patients reported improvement and 20 percent had complete recovery, approximately half were symptomatic for more than 30 years. Forty percent to 60 percent of patients improve with SSRIs, but most relapse within a month of discontinuing their medication.

The course of untreated social phobia is chronic, with an average duration of 20 years. Only 25 percent of patients spontaneously recover from the condition. When treated with either medications or cognitive-behavioral therapy, the response rate for uncomplicated social phobias is about 50 percent. If medications are stopped within three months, two-thirds of successfully treated patients relapse. Treatment for 6–12 months may decrease this relapse rate.

Summary

Anxiety, with or without autonomic hyperactivity, is a common complaint in primary care practice. Some anxious patients are appropriately worried about a threatening situation, such as poor health or a deteriorating relationship. Others seem apprehensive out of proportion to their circumstances, and most of these individuals are found to have an anxiety disorder, such as panic disorder or generalized anxiety disorder. Symptomatic treatment for anxiety is effective, and primary care physicians are able to provide the medication and supportive psychotherapy needed by many of their anxious patients. In severe or refractory cases, referral to a psychiatrist or other mental health practitioner is indicated. Because anxiety disorders tend to recur, primary care physicians should monitor their anxious patients for signs of relapse.

REFERENCES

American Psychiatric Association. Practice Guideline for the Treatment of Patients with Panic Disorder. *American Journal of Psychiatry* 155 (1998): May Supplement.

Davidson, Jonathan R. T. Pharmacotherapy of Social Anxiety Disorder. *Journal of Clinical Psychiatry* 59, suppl. 17 (1998): 47–51.

Flament, Martine F., and Bisserbe, Jean-Claude. Pharmacologic Treatment of Obsessive-Compulsive Disorder: Comparative Studies. *Journal of Clinical Psychiatry* 58, suppl. 12 (1997): 18–22.

Hales, Robert E.; Hilty, Donald A.; and Wise, Michael G. A Treatment Algorithm for the Management of Anxiety in Primary Care Practice. *Journal of Clinical Psychiatry* 58, suppl. 3 (1997): 76–80.

Hirschfeld, Robert M. A. Panic Disorder: Diagnosis, Epidemiology, and Clinical Course. *Journal of Clinical Psychiatry* 57, suppl. 10 (1996): 3–8.

Lieberman, Joseph A., III. BATHE: An Approach to the Interview Process in the Primary Care Setting. *Journal of Clinical Psychiatry* 58, suppl. 3 (1997): 3–6.

Rickels, Karl, and Schweizer, Edward. The Clinical Presentation of Generalized Anxiety in Primary-Care Settings: Practical Concepts of Classification and Management. *Journal of Clinical Psychiatry* 58, suppl. 11 (1997): 4–10.

Sherbourne, Cathy D.; Jackson, Catherine A.; Meredith, Lisa S.; Camp, Patti; and Wells, Kenneth B. Prevalence of Comorbid Anxiety Disorders in Primary Care Outpatients. *Archives of Family Medicine* 5 (1996): 27–34.

Skoog, Gunnar, and Skoog, Ingmar. A Forty-Year Follow-up of Patients with Obsessive-Compulsive Disorder. *Archives of General Psychiatry* 56 (1999): 121–127.

Spitzer, Robert L.; Williams, Janet B. W.; Kroenke, Kurt; Linzer, Mark; deGruy, Frank Verloin, III; Hahn, Steven R.; Brody, David; and Johnson, Jeffrey G. Utility of a New Procedure for Diagnosing Mental Disorders in Primary Care: The PRIME-MD 1000 Study. *Journal of the American Medical Association* 272 (1994): 1749–1756.

Stoudemire, Alan. Epidemiology and Psychopharmacology of Anxiety in Medical Patients. *Journal of Clinical Psychiatry* 57, suppl. 7 (1996): 64–72.

FOUR

Forgetfulness

Peter V. Rabins, M.D., M.P.H.

The complaint of forgetfulness is usually generated by family members. Less often it comes directly from the patient. Primary care physicians should suspect cognitive impairment if the patient is vague, is repetitive, or has forgotten prior interactions. Poor memory is by far the most common presenting symptom in people with cognitive impairment, but the chief complaint is sometimes low energy, sadness, change in behavior, or hallucinations, and only on examination does the physician identify the presence of cognitive dysfunction.

Syndromes of Cognitive Impairment

Decline in cognitive performance can be subdivided into three broad categories: delirium, dementia, and focal syndromes. In *delirium,* several areas of cognitive performance are deficient, but the distinguishing feature is an impairment in the level of consciousness. *Level of consciousness* refers to a patient's alertness, attentiveness, and ability to concentrate. A delirious individual is inattentive and therefore has difficulty remaining focused on a topic during conversation. Patients with delirium are usually drowsy and slowed down in thought and movement. Less commonly (as in delirium tremens), they appear very alert, tense, and restless and are overreactive to stimuli such as sound, light, or touch. Delirium usually has an acute or subacute onset, developing over hours or days. It often fluctuates in severity during the course of the day and is usually worse at night. Unpleasant moods (e.g., bewilderment, fear, sadness) and visual illusions and hallucinations are common.

Table 4.1. Comparison of Delirium, Dementia, and Focal Syndromes

Characteristic	Delirium	Dementia	Focal Syndrome
Onset	Usually acute	Usually gradual	Depends on etiology
Number of cognitive impairments	Multiple	Multiple	Single
Memory impairment	Almost always	Almost always	Only if amnestic syndrome
Level of consciousness	Altered	Normal	Normal
Associated symptoms			
Hallucinations and delusions	Very common	Common	Rare
Sleep-wake cycle	Often abnormal	Sometimes reversed	Intact
Depression	Common	Occasional	Rare

Dementia is characterized by multiple cognitive impairments and a normal level of consciousness. Memory is almost always affected. The pattern of deficits is often characteristic of a specific disorder (see below). Dementia usually develops gradually; by the time it comes to the attention of the physician, symptoms have generally been present for months or years.

Focal syndromes are conditions in which there is only a single cognitive deficit. When memory is the only dysfunction and the level of consciousness is normal, the condition is referred to as an *amnestic syndrome*. Other focal defects that may be present with complaints of forgetfulness or poor memory are *agnosia* (inability to recognize previously familiar objects, places, or people), *apraxia* (inability to carry out learned motor movements, such as writing or using eating utensils), and *aphasia* (inability to use language).

Table 4.1 compares the characteristics of delirium, dementia, and focal syndromes.

Common Causes of Forgetfulness

Delirium

Delirium is most commonly caused by metabolic derangements, infectious disorders, and hypoxia. The most frequent metabolic etiologies are electrolyte disturbances and organ failure (e.g., uremia). Of the drugs, anticholinergic compounds (e.g., tricyclic antidepressants, antihistamines, antispasmodics), narcotics, steroids, and antiparkinsonian agents (e.g., L-dopa, bromocriptine mesylate) are the chief culprits. Benzodiazepine, barbiturate, or alcohol intoxication also cause delirium, as can withdrawal from benzodiazepine, barbiturate, or alcohol. The physician should suspect alcohol, benzodiazepine, and/or barbiturate withdrawal in hospitalized patients when delirium (especially delirium tremens) develops several days after hospitalization and no other cause is identified.

Dementia

The most common cause of dementia is Alzheimer disease, which accounts for approximately 60 percent of cases. Alzheimer disease is a diagnosis of both inclusion and exclusion. Inclusion criteria are the gradual development of cognitive decline over months or years, impairments in memory, and at least one other cognitive dysfunction (i.e., aphasia, apraxia, or agnosia). The exclusion criterion is that other causes (e.g., cerebrovascular disease, Parkinson disease, major depression, hypothyroidism, pernicious anemia, subdural hematoma) have been ruled out.

Cerebrovascular disease is the second most common cause of dementia and accounts for 10–20 percent of cases. Unfortunately, valid diagnostic criteria have not been well established, and even expert clinicians are wrong about 50 percent of the time when making this diagnosis. The physician should suspect vascular dementia when the history suggests that cognitive deficits began suddenly; the physical examination identifies focal neurologic abnormalities, such as hemiparesis and reflex asymmetry; risk factors for cerebrovascular disease (e.g., hypertension, diabetes) are present; and an imaging study reveals strokelike lesions that correspond to the physical findings. In the past, overreliance on computed tomographic (CT) or magnetic resonance imaging (MRI) findings of white matter abnormalities led to an overdiagnosis of vascular dementia.

Dementia with Lewy bodies, which accounts for 5–10 percent of dementia, presents with parkinsonism, visual hallucinations, delusions, and memory impairment. Aphasia, apraxia, and agnosia are commonly present.

Frontal or frontotemporal degeneration (including Pick disease) causes approximately 5 percent of cases of dementia. Personality change, apathy, memory impairment, and aphasia are prominent early.

Dementia can be seen in many neurologic disorders that involve the brain. In Parkinson disease, for example, it eventually occurs in 30–60 percent of patients.

Potentially curable dementias are rare but should be considered. Chronic subdural hematoma, hydrocephalus (characterized by dementia, gait disorder, and incontinence), major depression, gradually developing renal failure, endocrinopathies (e.g., hypothyroidism, hyperparathyroidism), and chronic central nervous system (CNS) infection (e.g., human immunodeficiency virus [HIV], syphilis) can cause partially or fully reversible dementias.

Focal Syndromes

Focal syndromes can be caused by any disorder that damages isolated, strategic areas of the brain. Stroke, tumors, and abscesses are frequently responsible. Alcohol abuse with thiamine deficiency and idiopathic hippocampal sclerosis are the most common causes of amnestic (isolated memory loss) syndrome.

Assessment

Whenever the primary care physician suspects cognitive dysfunction, he or she should perform a cognitive mental status examination. Such an examination serves several purposes: it determines whether there is a deficit in cognitive performance, it identifies the aspects of cognition that are impaired, and it quantifies the degree of impairment. The evaluation should also include an assessment of noncognitive phenomena (e.g., mood, illusions, hallucinations, delusions) because a variety of psychiatric disorders can impair cognition and cause distress in the patient or caregiver, or both.

Chapter 1 discusses the Mini-Mental State Examination (MMSE) and suggests ways to determine the presence of abnormal mood, illusions, hallucinations, and delusions. A dementia due to major depression is often accompanied by delusions that are characteristic of depression, such as hypochondriacal beliefs (e.g., no bowel movements for many weeks without evidence of constipation), ideas of poverty (e.g., complaints of no money, insurance, or clothing when that is not the case), or guilt and self-blame (e.g., unfounded beliefs that the person has harmed others). Because depressed patients often feel unwell, with insomnia, anorexia, and lethargy, they may present to their primary care physicians with somatic complaints.

A thorough history and physical examination (including neurologic examination) should be carried out. This is important because most curable causes of dementia are revealed by their characteristic symptoms (e.g., cold intolerance in hypothyroidism) and signs (e.g., hyporeflexia).

A screening laboratory evaluation consists of a complete blood count (CBC), full chemistry panel, thyroid function tests, a serologic test for syphilis, and a B_{12} level. If the history or physical examination suggests a particular disorder, the physician should request appropriate tests. Thus, exposure to a heavy metal or the finding of a peripheral neuropathy indicates the need for a heavy-metal screen, and exposure to risk factors for HIV necessitates an HIV test.

Indications for head imaging are not well established. Several consensus conferences have concluded that a head-imaging study is not required in all cases of forgetfulness. I recommend that an imaging study be done when the history is of less than three years' duration, the patient is under the age of 70, the neurologic examination identifies a focal abnormality or suggests a specific syndrome (e.g., the gait disorder of hydrocephalus), or the cognitive examination reveals a focal syndrome. In most circumstances a noncontrast head CT is adequate. Many clinicians order a head MRI when they suspect vascular dementia, but the cost is approximately twice that of a CT scan.

A lumbar puncture should be performed after a head-imaging study has been done when the onset of illness is acute or subacute (hours to months), if the history or physical findings are compatible with meningitis or encephalitis, or when the serum fluorescent treponemal antibody (FTA) is positive. An electroencephalogram should be ordered when the level of consciousness is impaired (i.e., when delirium is suspected) or if a seizure disorder or Creutzfeldt-Jakob disease is in the differential diagnosis. The primary care physician should request neuropsychological testing when he or she is not sure whether a cognitive deficit is present, when symptoms are atypical, when the patient is young, or when clinical and laboratory findings do not point to a specific syndrome.

If the initial clinical assessment confirms that a cognitive impairment is present, the physician should inform the patient and any accompanying family members that he or she is concerned about the patient's memory. The physician should explain the planned laboratory and radiologic evaluations and schedule a follow-up appointment. The majority of patients with Alzheimer disease are unaware that they have a problem and often deny that their impairment is significant (e.g., "I know my memory is not so good, but that's true of everyone my age"). Trying to convince such individuals that they have an impairment when they adamantly deny it is usually unsuccessful. Therefore, I do not recommend confronting the patient with the diagnosis; I merely tell them that there are further tests to order. I sometimes give the family a prescription that states "Dr. Rabins ordered the following tests on February 10th" and suggest that the family show this if the patient resists.

Prognosis

Alzheimer disease lasts, on average, nine years, but autopsy-proven cases suggest the range is 3–22 years. Vascular dementia, dementia with Lewy bodies, and frontotemporal dementia result in shorter life expectancies than does Alzheimer disease.

Referral to Specialists

The primary care physician should consider referral to a neurologist, neuropsychiatrist, geriatric psychiatrist, or geriatrician when he or she suspects dementia and the patient is under 65, the neurologic examination suggests an uncommon syndrome, the history and physical examination are atypical, or management is complex because of coexisting medical and neurologic conditions. The physician should consider referral to a psychiatrist when a primary psychiatric disorder is a possible or likely cause of forgetfulness or when behavioral, emotional, or experiential (e.g., hallucinations, delusions) symptoms are prominent or unresponsive to therapy.

Case Example: A 68-year-old retired engineer reported to his physician at his annual examination that he was worried about his memory. He had mixed up the names of his grandchildren, missed an appointment to get his hair cut, and lost several strokes on his golf game. He continued to play bridge, however, to drive, and to do his taxes without problems. There was no change in appetite, sleep, or mood. Physical examination revealed no new abnormalities, mental status examination showed no evidence of depression, and the patient's MMSE score was 29/30 (he missed the date by one day). His physician concluded that there was no current evidence of dementia and informed the patient of this impression. He told him that referral to a specialist was unnecessary but would be arranged if the patient could not otherwise be reassured. The patient accepted the physician's formulation and agreed to a reassessment in six months.

In this case there was no objective evidence of significant cognitive impairment and no decline in function. The episodes of forgetfulness reported by the patient were minor and within the bounds of normal age-associated memory changes.

Case Example: A 64-year-old executive consulted her physician because of concerns about declining function at work. For the past several months, she had had difficulty following discussions similar to those she had led in the past, but she reported no other difficulties. History and physical examination showed no new problems since her last routine assessment 13 months before, and her mild hypertension was well controlled. On mental status examination there was no evidence of mood disorder and her MMSE score was 28/30, but on the latter test she missed the date by three days and could not copy the interlocking pentagons. Her physician initiated an evaluation for reversible causes of dementia and ordered a head MRI because of her young age. When these tests were normal, he referred her to a neuropsychiatrist for further differential diagnosis and to a neuropsychologist for more extensive cognitive assessment. Neuropsychological testing demonstrated deficits in memory, language, and visuospatial function. A diagnosis of possible Alzheimer disease was made.

In this case the patient reported cognitive impairments that were interfering with work. The MMSE and neuropsychological testing revealed visuospatial abnormalities that would be abnormal at any age. The history of progression over a number of months; normal neurologic examination, laboratory results, and imaging study; and the absence of evidence of stroke on either the neurologic examination or the imaging study pointed toward Alzheimer disease and away from vascular dementia. While the shorter time course would be compatible with rare conditions such as Creutzfeldt-Jakob disease, the lack of characteristic neurologic abnormalities (e.g., myoclonus) did not support that diagnosis.

The Treatment of Delirium

Once delirium is diagnosed, its causes can be sought and its manifestations treated. Common and important manifestations of delirium include disorientation, illusions, hallucinations, delusions, and agitation. Recommended interventions for disorientation include frequent reorientation, especially every time there is an interaction with the patient (e.g., "Hello, Mrs. Jones. I'm Dr. Smith. I'm glad to say that your heart failure is better and we expect your breathing to be better soon"); moderate levels of stimulation; and placement of wall calendars and clocks in the patient's room.

Illusions, hallucinations, and delusions are often frightening to patients and can lead to dangerous behavior. If they do not abate rapidly with reversal of the underlying cause of the delirium, they are best treated with neuroleptic drugs. Haloperidol, 0.5 mg po or im q2-4h, or risperidone, 0.5–1 mg po q4h, is often effective. Patients should be monitored for extrapyramidal side effects such as rigidity and tremor. Patients who are agitated or aggressive may require higher doses of neuroleptics or benefit from a fast-acting agent such as droperidol, 0.5–2 cc im, to initiate therapy. Benzodiazepines should be given when alcohol or benzodiazepine withdrawal is suspected, but they will not reverse hallucinations and delusions, as neuroleptics do. Parenterally administered short-acting benzodiazepines such as midazolam hydrochloride or intermediate-acting agents such as lorazepam are, however, useful for rapid sedation of delirious patients whose behavior is dangerous and for whom neuroleptics are risky. When parenteral neuroleptics or benzodiazepines are needed, constant observation and frequent monitoring of vital signs in an appropriate environment are indicated.

The Treatment of Dementia

The treatment of dementia focuses on three areas: cognitive symptoms, noncognitive symptoms, and family and other caregivers.

The Treatment of Cognitive Symptoms

Cholinesterase inhibitors are the most effective psychopharmacologic agents for enhancing cognition in Alzheimer disease. Tacrine hydrochloride is used only for patients who had significant improvement when the drug was first released and still appear to be benefiting from it. Donepezil hydrochloride is as effective as tacrine but is less likely to cause the gastrointestinal side effects and liver toxicity associated with the latter drug. The initial dose of donepezil is 5 mg po qhs, with an increase to 10 mg po qhs after one month. In clinical studies 50–65 percent of patients have a favorable response. There are no data on whether it is useful to continue the drug with individuals who do not show cognitive or functional improvement, how long the drug should be prescribed, or whether cholinesterase inhibitors are effective in late-stage Alzheimer disease. At 10 mg qhs, the monthly cost of donepezil is approximately $120. Discontinuation studies suggest that some individuals deteriorate when the drug is stopped. Clinical practice supports reinstituting the agent if this happens. Families should be cautioned that the average response is modest.

Other cholinergic-enhancing agents are likely to be approved by the Food and Drug Administration over the next several years. It will be difficult to determine the comparative efficacy of these agents, but it is unlikely that concomitant prescriptions of more than one cholinesterase inhibitor will be recommended.

Vitamin E, 2,000 IU po qd, and selegiline hydrochloride, 10 mg po qd, were found to delay nursing home placement and to slow functional decline in one large study. Cognition did not improve. There is not yet a consensus on the use of vitamin E, but many experts support its use because it is safe. Ginkgo biloba had a small beneficial effect on cognition in one study of individuals who had either Alzheimer disease or vascular dementia, but the magnitude of improvement seems to be less than that with cholinesterase inhibitors. Ginkgo has very few adverse effects. There are no published studies on the concomitant use of cholinesterase inhibitors, vitamin E, and ginkgo for cognitive enhancement.

The Treatment of Noncognitive Symptoms

Approximately two-thirds of patients with Alzheimer disease will experience a hallucination or delusion at some point in the illness. About 20 percent will have symptoms of major depression. Other common noncognitive symptoms include wandering, pacing, physical aggression, apathy, and sleep disturbance.

The treatment of these noncognitive symptoms should begin with a careful assessment. If the physician can identify a psychiatric syndrome such as major depression, then he or she should consider pharmacotherapy as an initial approach. More often, no specific psychiatric syndrome is identified, but particular behavior problems, such as not sleeping at night, physical overactivity, and verbal or physical threats directed toward others, are present. When this is the case, most experts recommend nonpharmacologic therapy as the first approach unless the behaviors are dangerous or causing significant distress to the patient or others.

The assessment of behavior disorder should include a careful evaluation of the environment and the patient's medical status. Disordered behavior may be precipitated by newly occurring delirium and by caregivers who are unaware of the patient's specific cognitive deficits. An example of the latter cause is that patients with Alzheimer disease who are asked to perform a task with multiple stages may be unable to comprehend the request because they are aphasic or unable to do it because they are apractic. The frustration that arises from the communication disorder or apraxia may lead to disruptive behavior. In this instance, the most appropriate treatment would be to inform those caring for the patient about that individual's limitations and to instruct them to modify their approach so that less is demanded of the patient. Structured activity programs are effective in decreasing undesirable behaviors in the nursing home setting, and this principle is likely to be true in day-care centers and at home as well.

Neuroleptic drugs are the mainstay of the pharmacotherapy of aggressive behaviors, hallucinations, and delusions. Because these drugs may cause adverse side effects (e.g., parkinsonism, rigidity with falls, tardive dyskinesia), the physician should clearly justify their use in the patient's chart. Most clinicians recommend the use of the newer, so-called atypical neuroleptics at low doses because they have fewer side effects. Typical starting doses are risperidone, 0.5 mg po qhs, or olanzapine, 2.5 mg po qd. These agents are expensive (e.g., at 2.5 mg qd, the monthly cost of olanzapine is approximately $150), however, and it is often possible to prescribe less-expensive drugs such as haloperidol, 0.5 mg po qd (monthly cost as low as $6), or thiothixene, 1 mg po qd (monthly cost as low as $10). In general, no more than 3 mg of risperidone, 10 mg of olanzapine, 4 mg of haloperidol, or 6 mg of thiothixene per day should be prescribed. When sleep disorder is present, the neuroleptic should be given all at night. Some physicians recommend spreading neuroleptic medication out through the day if the behavior disorder occurs intermittently or unpredictably, but no study has demonstrated the effectiveness of this approach.

In general, benzodiazepines are not recommended for the treatment of aggressive or disinhibited behavior. Their role in the treatment of concomitant anxiety is not clear. Recent small studies support the use of the anticonvulsants carbamazepine and divalproex sodium for the treatment of aggressive behavior. Buspirone hydrochloride and trazodone hydrochloride are occasionally beneficial in treating physical aggression. Trazodone, 50–100 mg po qhs, can be used for isolated sleep disorder.

Case Example: A 76-year-old man came for his annual checkup accompanied by his wife. She reported having been worried about his memory for several years. When asked to elaborate, she said that he repeated himself frequently, had been more irritable, and had been unable to complete their tax forms despite having done them for many years. On one occasion, when they were waiting in line for symphony tickets, he inexplicably began yelling. The patient had well-controlled adult-onset diabetes and a left bundle branch block. Physical examination was notable only for mild peripheral neuropathy. On mental status examination, the patient had no awareness that he had memory and behavioral difficulties. MMSE score was 19/30, with impairments in memory (disorientation and poor recall), language (inability to repeat a phrase correctly), attention and concentration (difficulty subtracting serial sevens), and visuospatial performance (inability to copy interlocking pentagons). Blood tests for reversible causes of dementia and a head CT were unrevealing.

The physician made a diagnosis of probable Alzheimer disease. The history extending back at least two years, gradual progression without focal neurologic abnormalities, and a cognitive examination that demonstrated impairments in memory, language, visuospatial performance, and initiative all supported this diagnosis. A cholinesterase inhibitor, donepezil, was started at a dose of 5 mg po qhs.

On follow-up, the patient's MMSE score had improved by only one point, but his wife reported that he was repeating himself less and seemed more able to help around the kitchen. Based on these improvements, the physician decided to continue the drug. The patient's occasional emotional outbursts were thought to be "catastrophic reactions" (i.e., distressing emotional responses to circumstances in which he could not overcome his cognitive impairments). The patient's wife was taught that these reactions could be minimized by trying to avoid overwhelming situations. She was also referred to the Alzheimer Association, and she found their support groups helpful.

In this case, the diagnosis of probable Alzheimer disease seems appropriate. There seemed to be functional improvement with a cholinesterase inhibitor even though cognitive testing was unchanged. The family chose to continue donepezil based on this possible improvement, and the physician increased the dose to 10 mg qhs.

Support and Treatment of the Caregiver

Demoralization and depression are present in 40–50 percent of caregivers of individuals with dementia. Some caregivers benefit from educational material or focused discussions on specific symptoms, treatments, and prognoses. Others may benefit from referral to support groups, such as those directed by the Alzheimer Association. (Local telephone numbers can be obtained by calling the Alzheimer Association at 1-800-272-3900.) Well-designed intervention trials demonstrate that a combination of emotional support and educational information benefit caregivers and that such programs can delay nursing home placement for the individuals they look after. When caregivers feel overwhelmed or demoralized despite such measures, the primary care physician should recommend counseling. If the dysphoric state persists despite psychotherapy, psychiatric referral is indicated, for the caregiver's distress may reflect not only the burden he or she bears, but also the presence of major depression or an anxiety disorder.

The Treatment of Focal Syndromes

The treatment of patients with isolated memory impairments (amnestic syndrome) includes searching for an etiology and ensuring safety. If alcohol abuse or thiamine deficiency is possible, the physician should prescribe thiamine, 100 mg im followed by 100 mg po qd. If alcohol abuse or thiamine deficiency is unlikely, cerebrovascular disease may be present and, if identified, should be treated appropriately. About 50 percent of patients who present with isolated memory impairment progress to a dementia syndrome within two years. Patients with aphasia should be referred for speech therapy. Otherwise, patients with focal syndromes should be treated using the general principles described under the treatment of dementia.

Patients Who Complain of Forgetfulness but for Whom No Disorder Is Identified

Eighty-five percent of individuals over 65 report that their memory is not as good as it was when they were younger. Empirical research demonstrates that this assertion is accurate. For most individuals, "forgetfulness" consists of difficulty coming up with names or words or occasionally misplacing keys and other objects. If no other cause for concern is present (e.g., becoming lost in familiar surroundings or losing a skill such as cooking or balancing a checkbook) and a cognitive examination identifies no problems, reassurance with reassessment in six months is appropriate.

Elderly patients frequently ask whether physical or intellectual activity prevents cognitive decline. There is no evidence that this is the case, but there is a small research literature suggesting that individuals who use mnemonics and memory aids, such as writing down important information, and who are taught to worry less about their memory perform better on repeated cognitive testing. Primary care physicians can help older individuals who are concerned about their memory but have no evidence of dementia by passing along this information and encouraging them to remain physically and intellectually active as part of a healthy lifestyle.

Summary

Declining cognition can be classified as *delirium,* a syndrome in which multiple cognitive impairments occur in the setting of an altered level of consciousness; *focal syndromes,* in which only a single area of cognitive function has deteriorated; or *dementia,* in which multiple areas of cognition have declined in the presence of a normal level of consciousness. After the physician decides which of these syndromes is present, he or she can use a specific algorithm to discover its etiology. Delirium is most commonly due to an acute toxic or metabolic process, although many other conditions can cause the syndrome. Dementia is most commonly due to Alzheimer disease or cerebrovascular disease, while focal syndromes are generally caused by single brain lesions. The most effective treatments are those directed to the underlying pathological process. When such treatment cannot be done, symptoms and signs are the focus of care. Even in the face of irreversible structural brain disease, clinical improvement is often possible.

REFERENCES

American Psychiatric Association. Practice Guideline for the Treatment of Patients with Alzheimer's Disease and Other Dementias of Late Life. *American Journal of Psychiatry* 154 (1997): May Supplement.

LeBars, Pierre L.; Katz, Martin M.; Berman, Nancy; Itil, Turan M.; Freedman, Alfred M.; and Schatzberg, Alan F. A Placebo-Controlled, Double-Blind, Randomized Trial of an Extract of Ginkgo Biloba for Dementia. *Journal of the American Medical Association* 278 (1997): 1327–1332.

Mace, Nancy L., and Rabins, Peter V. *The 36-Hour Day: A Family Guide to Caring for Persons with Alzheimer Disease, Related Dementing Illnesses, and Memory Loss in Later Life,* 3d ed. Baltimore: Johns Hopkins University Press, 1999.

Mittelman, Mary S.; Ferris, Steven H.; Shulman, Emma; Steinberg, Gertrude; and Levin, Bruce. A Family Intervention to Delay Nursing Home Placement of Patients with

Alzheimer Disease: A Randomized Controlled Trial. *Journal of the American Medical Association* 276 (1996): 1725–1731.

Sano, Mary; Ernesto, Christopher; Thomas, Ronald G.; Klauber, Melville R.; Schafer, Kimberly; Grundman, Michael; Woodbury, Peter; Growdon, John; Cotman, Carl W.; Pfeiffer, Eric; Schneider, Lon S.; and Thal, Leon J. A Controlled Trial of Selegiline, Alpha-Tocopherol, or Both as Treatment for Alzheimer's Disease. *New England Journal of Medicine* 336 (1997): 1216–1222.

Schneider, Lon S.; Pollock, Vicki E.; and Lyness, Scott A. A Meta-analysis of Controlled Trials of Neuroleptic Treatment in Dementia. *Journal of the American Geriatrics Society* 38 (1990): 553–563.

Slavney, Phillip R. *Psychiatric Dimensions of Medical Practice: What Primary-Care Physicians Should Know about Delirium, Demoralization, Suicidal Thinking, and Competence to Refuse Medical Advice.* Baltimore: Johns Hopkins University Press, 1998.

FIVE

Unrealistic Concerns about Health

Mark L. Teitelbaum, M.D.

Patients who cannot be reassured about their health are some of the most difficult for physicians. Because such patients have somatic complaints that are medically unexplained despite adequate investigation, patients and physicians may be at odds over what the symptoms indicate. Further, some of these patients may insist on surgery, be dependent on narcotics, or threaten lawsuits. Physicians commonly use terms such as *psychogenic, functional, psychosomatic, hysterical,* or *hypochondriacal* to describe the complaints or the patients themselves. Sometimes, these labels are used in a pejorative way. This is unfortunate because the patients are genuinely suffering and in need of help.

Epidemiology

Somatic symptoms are extremely common. It has been estimated that 60–80 percent of a normal population experience one physical symptom per week and that anywhere from 20 percent to 80 percent of patients presenting to primary care physicians have poorly explained somatic complaints. Culture, personality, and gender may all be predisposing factors in generating unexplained medical complaints. Female sex may be influential in three ways: (1) women report more symptoms in general than men do, (2) women visit physicians more often than men do, and (3) the two most common psychiatric disorders that present with prominent somatic symptoms (i.e., major depression and anxiety disorders) occur more frequently in women than in men.

General Clinical Features

Patients who cannot be reassured about their health are preoccupied with one or more usually persistent but often ill-defined problems on which a concern about disease rests. Pain, fatigue, weakness, vague neurologic symptoms, and gastrointestinal distress are common complaints. The patient may also report growing difficulty in work, social functioning, and family relationships, all of which have deteriorated. The patient's history often includes excessive spending of money, time, and energy on visiting a variety of physicians and hospitals in search of help. The patient may also describe a growing sense of discouragement that the bodily source of the illness will ever be discovered.

Differential Diagnosis

The differential diagnosis of medically unexplained complaints includes six conditions.

— Unrecognized medical disorders
— Major depression
— Anxiety disorders
— Conversion disorder
— Somatization disorder
— Schizophrenia and delusional disorder, somatic type

Unrecognized Medical Disorders

Medical disorders presenting with vague symptoms include conditions such as multiple sclerosis, systemic lupus erythematosus, myasthenia gravis, and hypothyroidism. One study involving long-term follow-up of patients with physical symptoms thought to be "hysterical" showed that about one-third were subsequently discovered to have a physical disorder, unrecognized at the time of initial presentation.

Major Depression

Physical complaints are very common in major depression. Lack of energy, gastrointestinal symptoms, anorexia, weight loss, sexual dysfunction, and vague pains or headache may be the patient's chief complaint. Typical findings of a low mood, poor self-esteem, feelings of hopelessness, suicidal thoughts, and signs of slowed psychomotor activity support the diagnosis of major depression. Some patients have a delusional belief that they have cancer, AIDS, or another terrible disease. There may be previous episodes of depression or mania and a family history of affective disorder. It is not understood why some patients with major depression present to physicians with primarily physical complaints while others do not. The former patients may have different premorbid personalities (e.g., more introverted), have had different early life experiences (e.g., more losses), or be products of a different sociocultural environment (e.g., a culture that disapproves of emotional expression). The prevalence of major depression in primary care settings is about 5 percent.

> *Case Example:* A married, middle-aged business executive was admitted to the hospital because of fatigue and weakness of six months' duration. A thorough medical evaluation was unremarkable. A psychiatric evaluation revealed an ambitious, hard-driving, and energetic man who was quite successful in his work. He described himself as "functioning ineffectively and thinking inefficiently" of late, yet he denied feeling sad. He stated that he simply felt "disappointed" in himself and described a feeling of hopelessness about his chances of recovery despite the fact that no serious physical disorder had been diagnosed. Along with his lowered energy and vitality, he described significant changes in his appetite and sex drive. His overall enjoyment of life was diminished. Examination of his mental state also revealed psychomotor retardation. Formal cognitive testing was entirely within normal limits. The diagnosis of major depression was made.

Anxiety Disorders

Patients with anxiety disorders who are seen in the primary care setting frequently present with somatic complaints such as chest pain, palpitations, dyspnea, weakness, lightheadedness, dizziness, vertigo, tremor, diarrhea, or vomiting. Findings of tenseness, apprehension, or worry—sometimes associated with difficulty concentrating, insomnia, and fatigue—suggest the existence of an anxiety disorder. Some patients may give a history of panic attacks associated with fear of impending death accompanied by signs of sympathetic nervous system arousal. Other patients may report fears of being alone or leaving their homes and may have become housebound as a result of their illness. The prevalence of anxiety disorders in primary care settings is about 7 percent.

> *Case Example:* A married, middle-aged woman was hospitalized to evaluate leg weakness and fear of walking for about two years. Her illness had begun acutely, within days after her mother's unexpected death. At that time she had been alone in her house while her husband was away on business. She was awakened suddenly from sleep with palpitations, dyspnea, lightheadedness, weakness in her legs, and an overwhelming sense of terror and impending death. She called her family physician, who came to her home, recognized her state of panic, and gave her an injection of a sedative medication. He told her to stay in bed until she felt better. The patient described falling asleep quickly after the injection. On waking the next day, she attempted to get out of bed, but once again felt weak, lightheaded, and fearful. Her legs collapsed under her, and she got back into bed, where she remained. When her husband returned home the next day, he found her in bed, afraid to get up and fearful that she would "feel weak and fall." A series of hospitalizations with negative evaluations occurred over the next two years, during which the patient spent most of her time in bed or in her swimming pool. She was reluctant to walk or go out of her house alone, and almost every attempt to do so precipitated a recurrence of symptoms identical to the original attack. Her illness required her husband to change his job so he could care for her. An extensive medical workup was again negative.
>
> Psychiatric evaluation led to the conclusion that the patient had panic disorder with agoraphobia. Her refusal to walk or go out alone was understood as being related to her fears of having an attack with no one there to help.

"Hysteria"

Patients with "hysterical" complaints behave as if they have a somatic disorder when they do not. The behavior is undertaken to get attention, affection, or compensation; to obtain relief from guilt or other unpleasant affects;

to avoid responsibility; or to solve some other life difficulty. The goal of the behavior is generally outside the patient's awareness, which distinguishes "hysteria" from factitious disease and malingering.

Conversion Disorder (Acute "Hysteria"). "Hysterical" behavior may begin abruptly in the setting of a stressful situation such as a deteriorating marriage, an unpleasant job, a motor vehicle accident, combat, or bereavement. The nature of the patient's complaint may involve the unconscious copying of an illness previously experienced by a family member or other person known or seen by the patient. The complaint may also convey something about the meaning of the person's distress, which is symbolically communicated through "body language." The diagnosis ultimately rests on recognizing (1) a vulnerable personality, often with self-dramatizing, passive, or immature features; (2) a situation understood as stressful and disruptive to the person involved; (3) symptoms or signs unexplained by physiologic processes; and (4) the purpose the behavior serves in solving a life problem.

> *Case Example:* A single young man was hospitalized with a one-month history of weakness of his legs and difficulty walking. Neurologic evaluation was unremarkable, yet the patient persisted in a fearful worry that he had multiple sclerosis. His present illness had started acutely, after he had begun a new job where he felt fearful of his boss, who was critical and demanding. The "final straw" came after he had begun dating a woman from his office. Although he saw their relationship as casual and platonic, she had begun pressing him for more of a commitment. After a distressing discussion with her one night, he awoke the next morning feeling weak in his legs and unable to walk. By temperament he was a dramatic, perfectionistic, and self-centered person. Examination of the patient's mental state did not reveal evidence of major depression, an anxiety disorder, or schizophrenia. His behavior was understood as motivated by both fears of dealing with situations he wished to avoid and a desire to "save face" at the same time. Being ill seemed to serve the purpose of keeping the patient from having to "stand up" up to his boss and "take steps" toward marriage without having to deal directly with either his boss or his girlfriend. A diagnosis of conversion disorder was made.

Somatization Disorder (Chronic "Hysteria"). Some patients with "hysterical" illnesses have long histories of many unexplained physical complaints involving multiple organ systems, usually starting in adolescence or young adulthood with exacerbations and remissions throughout life. Such patients may be taking unneeded medications (including narcotics) and have had numerous surgical procedures. Many have associated emotional disturbance or personality disorder with both self-dramatizing and self-doubting, perfectionistic features. Long-term follow-up of such patients has shown that in 90 percent of cases no new medical or psychiatric illness will appear within six to eight years of diagnosis. The prevalence of somatization disorder in primary care settings may be as high as 5 percent.

Case Example: A divorced, middle-aged woman was hospitalized with recurrent, vague abdominal pain. She had had poorly explained abdominal complaints since adolescence and her first surgery, an appendectomy, as a teenager. Over the years she had been operated on many times for unexplained pain and more recently for intestinal obstruction due to adhesions from previous surgeries. Her gallbladder, as well as portions of her stomach and small and large intestines, had been removed, all without pathological findings. She was taking a variety of medications, including tranquilizers and narcotics.

A psychiatric evaluation revealed a woman who seemed in no distress and did not look ill, though she said she had been ill all her life. The patient had grown up in a home with marital discord and described her mother as "cold and distant," her father as "loving." His death, approximately 10 years before, had occurred just before a marked increase in all her complaints and a downhill course that involved multiple hospitalizations and surgeries. Although she was now divorced, she remained locked in an emotional battle with her ex-husband.

The patient's preoccupation with her symptoms and her emotional withdrawal from her family were major factors in the failure of her marriage and her alienation from her children, who refused to visit her in hospital. She felt discouraged, lonely, and "hurt." Examination of the patient's mental state did not reveal symptoms of depressive illness. It did illuminate, however, her anger with her ex-husband and children for abandoning her, as well as her rage at several previous physicians who "didn't care." Furthermore, she reported multiple unexplained bodily complaints involving several organ systems. Her behavior was understood as motivated by a desire for love, care, and attention from others, which she could not ask for directly. A diagnosis of somatization disorder was made.

Schizophrenia and Delusional Disorder, Somatic Type

In schizophrenia, the patient's complaints center around a delusional belief of ill health. Unlike anxious patients who are fearful of illness, delusional patients (whether with schizophrenia, delusional disorder, or major depression) are convinced they are ill, often with a bizarre or unusual infestation, poisoning, metabolic derangement, or physical malformation. The diagnosis of schizophrenia is suggested by a history of previous episodes of hallucinations or delusions in clear consciousness and by the absence of evidence of coarse brain disease or major depression. The prevalence of schizophrenia in primary care settings is less than 1 percent.

> *Case Example:* A single, middle-aged woman was hospitalized with infected excoriations that covered a good deal of her skin. She admitted to almost continuous scratching because of generalized pruritus. The patient seemed "strange" to her physician, who could find no primary medical or dermatologic disorder to explain her complaint. It seemed that her scratching had produced the skin lesions, which then itched and provoked more scratching.
>
> A psychiatric evaluation revealed a disheveled woman who admitted to several psychiatric admissions "because of voices" since her early twenties. Examination of her mental state revealed the delusional belief that her itching was caused by "small worms" that had infiltrated her skin. She scratched some skin debris from her arm and gave it to the psychiatrist, saying, "Send this to the lab; you'll see them!" Informing the patient that skin biopsy examinations had been done and were negative was to no avail. A diagnosis of schizophrenia was made.

Psychiatric Consultation

The primary care physician should consider psychiatric consultation for all patients with poorly explained physical complaints who cannot be reassured about their health. The purpose of consultation is to help with the diagnostic process and planning for treatment. Preparing patients for consultation is important but often overlooked. The crucial elements in effective preparation are a full and open discussion with the patient of the physician's reason for requesting the consultation and the provision of enough time to listen for and deal with the patient's reactions.

Psychiatric consultation has a variety of meanings for patients that may lead them to reject the proposal, at least initially. Although idiosyncratic issues (e.g., a previous negative experience with a psychiatrist) are sometimes involved, certain common themes tend to recur.

Stigma

A patient may experience the recommendation for psychiatric consultation as an insult. Additionally, the patient may fear the physician's or another significant person's disapproval should a psychiatric disorder be diagnosed. In some instances, the patient is responding to a realistic perception of the physician's attitude toward psychiatric disorder and psychiatric patients. The physician can express positive regard for the patient and support the latter's self-esteem by conveying an empathic understanding of the patient's dilemma. When, for example, the patient is distressed by the proposal of a consultation, the primary care physician might say: "I'm sorry you're upset by my suggesting you see a psychiatrist. I'm concerned about you, and I want you to feel better. I know that sometimes complaints like yours can be due to emotional troubles or stressful circumstances, and you owe it to yourself to have that possibility checked out." Acceptance of a consultation is more likely when the patient feels respected and understood.

Abandonment

A patient may experience the recommendation for psychiatric consultation as an abandonment. Some patients are extremely sensitive to rejection and will resist psychiatric consultation because they feel that their relationship with their primary care physician is being threatened. Occasionally, patients may be responding to a realistic perception that the physician is wanting to withdraw from their care. It is helpful for the physician to reassure the patient that their relationship will continue, regardless of the recommendations the psychiatrist makes.

Depreciated Suffering

A patient may experience the recommendation for psychiatric consultation as being based on the primary care physician's belief that the symptoms are "imaginary" or "all in the head" or that the patient is not really suffering. Because such patients feel betrayed and lose trust in the physician, the latter should convey an appreciation of the reality of the patient's suffering. To diminish the likelihood of this type of reaction, the physician might say: "I know you are suffering greatly with your [pain, nausea, weakness]. The purpose of a psychiatric consultation is to explore all possible causes of your illness because emotional troubles and stressful circumstances can cause symptoms such as yours and produce real suffering. I want to find out what is causing the problem and help you do something about it."

Hopelessness

Patients may experience the recommendation for psychiatric consultation as a communication that their condition is hopeless, that nothing can be done, and that the referral to a psychiatrist is basically an "end of the line" or "last ditch" attempt to help. The inclusion of psychiatric consultation as an integral part of the evaluation as soon as the possibility of psychiatric disorder is suspected may work to mitigate against this sense of hopelessness. The physician can share a sense of realistic pessimism with the patient but should combat the unrealistic aspects of the patient's discouragement. For example, the physician might comment: "I share your pessimism about [discovering a neurologic cause for your symptoms, curing your pain with more surgery], but I don't share your hopelessness about getting well. It's very possible that psychiatric consultation may lead to a recommendation for treatment that could prove to be helpful."

Disappointment

A patient may react to the recommendation for psychiatric consultation with disappointment and loss of confidence in the primary care physician. Perhaps the physician is not very competent if he or she must ask for help.

A simple acknowledgment of the patient's disappointment can rekindle the patient's faith in the primary care physician, not as an all-knowing parental figure, but as a more realistically perceived, competent, insightful, and caring professional. The physician might comment that "everyone needs help sometimes, both doctors and patients alike!" Most patients are grateful to their physicians for requesting psychiatric consultation, and the primary physician-patient relationship is usually strengthened, not undermined.

Treatment

Presentation of the Diagnosis and Treatment Plan to the Patient

If a psychiatric disorder is diagnosed after thorough workup of a patient with unexplained physical complaints, the first step is the presentation to the patient of the diagnosis and its implications for treatment. This is usually done by the primary care physician, sometimes together with the consulting psychiatrist. It may be of help to have family members present when this summing up takes place, to avoid any miscommunication. The physician should explain that the patient's complaints do, indeed, have a cause: stress, anxiety, depression, or whatever term is most accurate and acceptable to the patient. The physician may wish to reiterate that there is no doubt of the patient's suffering despite the absence of a medical or surgical disorder to explain it. Many patients with psychiatric disorders who initially cannot be reassured about their health are best treated by their own physicians.

Treatment of the Underlying Psychiatric Disorder by the Patient's Physician

The treatment of conversion disorder and somatization disorder usually proceeds best if the physician sees the patient at regular intervals. Appointments on an as-needed basis tend to encourage an escalation of symptoms and should be avoided. The physician's aim is to encourage the patient to talk about personal difficulties while discouraging a focus on physical complaints. As a therapeutic alliance is created and trust established, the task may become progressively easier. Opportunities then arise to address the difficulties that are prompting maladaptive behavior and to search for more direct and satisfying solutions. For example, the physician may advise the patient on how to deal better with a work-related problem or may recommend counseling for a troubled marital relationship. Patients with conversion disorder and somatization disorder are often resistant to such undertakings or to psychiatric consultation. In these difficult cases, a stable physician-patient relationship and the elimination of doctor shopping and unneeded drugs, tests, and procedures are more realistic goals.

The treatment of depression and anxiety generally requires medications, suggestions for which are found in Chapters 2 and 3. The treatment of schizophrenia and delusional disorders is best undertaken by a psychiatrist, at least initially.

The Importance of Collaboration

When the primary care physician refers the patient to a psychiatrist for treatment, he or she should always make provision for ongoing general medical follow-up. The reasons for this are several. First of all, disrupting the primary physician-patient relationship will, in many instances, be a great loss to a patient who has counted on his or her physician over the years. Second, patients diagnosed as "hysterical" when first seen may subsequently be discovered to have medical disorders. Last, since psychiatric disorders and medical disorders seem to be associated at a frequency greater than chance, some patients with a psychiatric disorder presenting with physical complaints are probably at greater risk than nonpsychiatrically ill patients for becoming medically ill in the future. For collaboration to work, lines of communication between the psychiatrist and the primary care physician should be maintained. The latter should be aware that, during the course of psychiatric treatment, especially in its early stages, there are often crises during which the patient may wish to discontinue treatment and return to doctor shopping. The primary care physician can be of help during these periods in supporting the patient's continued efforts at psychiatric treatment and discouraging a renewed search for medical disease.

Limitation of Doctor Shopping

Limitation of doctor shopping is an important goal of treatment for a patient with medically unexplained physical complaints. Both the psychiatrist and the primary care physician should make every effort to persuade the patient to limit the number of doctors consulted.

Limitation of Unneeded Diagnostic Tests, Procedures, and Treatments

The limitation of unneeded diagnostic tests, procedures, and treatments is often difficult. The physician should consider additional testing only with the appearance of new signs (rather than symptoms) and should carefully limit testing. The physician should also avoid potentially harmful treatments and should recommend narcotics, sedatives, or surgery only when absolutely necessary. If there is a good physician-patient relationship, firm but kind limit setting is generally tolerated well.

Treatment by the Psychiatrist with Medical Follow-up

The psychiatrist might recommend treatment on an inpatient basis. This is needed for severe depressions with suicidal thinking and is often necessary for schizophrenia with delusions and for "hysteria" when the patient's behavior involves falling or an inability to walk or is associated with drug dependence and a need for detoxification. After discharge, such patients often need continued treatment by the psychiatrist with medical follow-up provided by the primary care physician.

Prognosis

Prognosis depends on the underlying condition discovered. With appropriate treatment, the outlook for recovery from major depression, anxiety disorders, and conversion disorder is good. The prognosis for patients with somatization disorder or schizophrenia is considerably more guarded.

Summary

Patients who cannot be reassured about their health are commonly encountered in primary care settings. The majority of these patients suffer from psychiatric illnesses, such as major depression, anxiety disorders, conversion disorder, somatization disorder, schizophrenia, or delusional disorder, somatic type. Primary care physicians should consider psychiatric consultation for all patients with poorly explained physical complaints who cannot be reassured about their health. Patients who reject a consultation initially can usually be persuaded to go ahead. If ongoing psychiatric treatment is needed, collaboration between the primary care physician and the psychiatrist is important.

REFERENCES

Bursztajn, Harold, and Barsky, Arthur J. Facilitating Patient Acceptance of a Psychiatric Referral. *Archives of Internal Medicine* 145 (1985): 73–75.

Lazare, Aaron. Current Concepts in Psychiatry: Conversion Symptoms. *New England Journal of Medicine* 305 (1981): 745–748.

Monson, Roberta A., and Smith, G. Richard, Jr. Current Concepts in Psychiatry: Somatization Disorder in Primary Care. *New England Journal of Medicine* 308 (1983): 1464–1465.

Slater, Eliot T. O., and Glithero, E. A Follow-up of Patients Diagnosed as Suffering from "Hysteria." *Journal of Psychosomatic Research* 9 (1965): 9–13.

Von Korff, Michael; Shapiro, Sam; Burke, Jack D.; Teitelbaum, Mark; Skinner, Elizabeth A.; German, Pearl; Turner, Raymond W.; Klein, Lawrence; and Burns, Barbara. Anxiety and Depression in a Primary Care Clinic: Comparison of Diagnostic Interview Schedule, General Health Questionnaire, and Practitioner Assessments. *Archives of General Psychiatry* 44 (1987): 152–156.

Wool, Carol A., and Barsky, Arthur J. Do Women Somatize More than Men? Gender Differences in Somatization. *Psychosomatics* 35 (1994): 445–452.

SIX

Suicidal Thoughts

Dean F. MacKinnon, M.D.

People who commit suicide have often seen a physician in the weeks before their death. During these visits it is unlikely that the patient raised the topic of suicide or that the physician asked about it. How, then, can physicians do a better job of recognizing potentially suicidal individuals? The first thing to understand is that suicide is associated with several risk factors.

Epidemiology

The Demographics of Suicide

Suicide is the ninth leading cause of death in the United States, with an annual rate of some 11 per 100,000. Over all age groups, men kill themselves more often than women and Caucasians more often than persons of other races. In people age 15–24, suicide is the third leading cause of death.

Caucasian males account for 75 percent of suicides in the United States. Although Caucasian women have much the same rates (2–5/100,000) across all age groups, Caucasian men are more likely to commit suicide the older they get: at age 60 the rate is 20/100,000; at age 85 it is 70/100,000.

Unmarried individuals are more likely to kill themselves than married ones, and Protestants more likely than Catholics and Jews.

Means Used to Commit Suicide

Firearms are by far the leading means of suicide fatality, with poisoning (including drug overdose) and suffocation (including hanging and carbon monoxide inhalation) next. Many "accidental" deaths in the form of motor vehicle crashes, falls, or drowning may be undocumented suicides.

Males are four times as likely as females to die by suicide, but females are twice as likely to attempt it. Women may attempt suicide more often because they have a higher rate of major depressive disorder; they may succeed less often because they tend to use less lethal means.

Suicide and Psychiatric Disorders

When investigators in different countries examine the medical records and interview the family and friends of people who have died by suicide, they find the same result: almost everyone who commits suicide had signs of a psychiatric disorder, and about half had sought psychiatric help in the past. The posthumous diagnoses most often are affective disorders (major depression or bipolar disorder), substance abuse disorders, personality disorders, and schizophrenia. At least two-thirds of persons who committed suicide had symptoms of major depression before death.

Clinical and community studies reveal that patients with psychiatric disorders have a remarkably high lifetime risk of completed suicide. Major depression has been associated with a 15–20 percent rate of completed suicide in follow-up of hospitalized patients (who are at higher risk for suicide because suicidal thought and self-injurious behavior are strong indications for hospitalization). Individuals with depression diagnosed in community surveys have a 5 percent lifetime risk of completed suicide (about 500 times the general population rate in the United States). Alcoholism and schizophrenia are associated with lifetime suicide rates in the 15–20 percent range.

Suicide and Medical Disorders

Medical disorders associated with an elevated risk of suicide are AIDS, cancer (especially head and neck), Huntington disease, multiple sclerosis, peptic ulcer disease, end-stage renal disease, spinal cord injury, and systemic lupus erythematosus. Any serious medical illness can raise the risk of suicide in elderly Caucasian men. In most cases, suicide in the context of a medical disorder occurs in conjunction with a depressive disorder or a history of alcohol abuse, or both.

Arguments by the assisted-suicide movement notwithstanding, the majority of patients with chronic or terminal medical disorders would prefer to struggle against death rather than bring it on themselves.

A Problem for Primary Care Physicians

Many physicians are hesitant to ask about suicidal thoughts, even as they prescribe antidepressant, anxiolytic, or hypnotic medications. Patients with suicidal thoughts rarely disclose them spontaneously, but almost all readily acknowledge them, once asked.

Screening for Suicidal Thoughts

The first challenge in helping patients who are thinking of suicide is usually to discover that they are having such thoughts. Patients are often reluctant to admit they are suicidal out of shame, stoicism, or fear of being regarded as "crazy." It is not practical or necessary to question every patient about suicidal thinking, but all patients who acknowledge depressive symptoms should be asked.

If a patient complains of or assents to feelings of sadness, loss, hopelessness, anger, or any other overwhelming, painful emotion, the physician should inquire about suicidal thoughts. If a patient complains of insomnia, loss of appetite or weight, lack of energy, or problems with memory and concentration, the primary care physician should ask about depressive moods, feelings of hopelessness, and suicidal thinking.

Certain other clinical situations raise the risk of suicide and thus lower the threshold for asking about it. At some point in the course of a patient's debilitating or terminal illness, the primary care physician should query the patient about low mood and thoughts of ending his or her life. The physician should also ask patients who have recently lost a spouse or young child. Depression or demoralization may be suspected when a patient is slow to recover function after a stroke, a heart attack, a fracture, or a limb amputation, and questions about mood and suicidal thoughts are indicated.

A patient who is not thinking about suicide will simply answer "No" when asked about it. A patient with suicidal thoughts will generally welcome the opportunity to discuss them. No patient is going to begin contemplating suicide just because a physician has asked about it. That being said, a tactful approach is more likely than a blunt one to elicit an honest answer. A physician can introduce the topic of suicide in several ways: "Some patients with feelings similar to yours have thoughts of ending their lives. Have you been having thoughts of that sort?" "Has your situation gotten so bad that you've thought of ending your life?" "Since you began having these feelings, have you also had thoughts of suicide?"

Family Informants

When a physician detects or suspects suicidal thoughts, he or she should almost always seek further information from family members. Patients and their relatives will benefit not only by working together to lessen the risk of suicide, but also by helping the physician make correct judgments about diagnosis, prognosis, and the need for emergency treatment. If a family member is in the waiting room, ask the patient if that person can be included in the discussion of suicidal thoughts or self-injurious behavior. If a relative is available but not present, ask that person to come into the office while the patient waits, or discuss the situation on the telephone with the patient in the room. Confidentiality should be preserved when possible, but if a potential for suicide exists, safety takes precedence.

When speaking with a patient's relative, try to confirm the patient's suicidal thoughts or self-injurious behavior without at first revealing details. A family member may thus be asked: "Have you been worried about [the patient]'s mood? Has [the patient] said or done anything that made you concerned about [the patient]'s safety?" Although many relatives of patients contemplating suicide will have been very uneasy and will welcome an opportunity to talk about it, sometimes they are unaware of the problem. In the latter case, the physician should break confidentiality and reveal the patient's potential for suicide. It is not possible to be forgiven by a corpse.

Assessing Suicidal Risk in Particular Situations

Patients Who Have Already Injured Themselves

■ *A patient comes to clinic Monday morning, referred by an emergency room physician, to report a suicide attempt over the weekend.*

■ *A spouse takes the physician aside to whisper that the patient did not accidentally drop the contents of his prescription in the toilet last week, as reported, but took them all at once.*

■ *A frantic parent discovers scratch marks on a teenager's wrist and wants to know what to do.*

The history of the self-injurious event usually provides important details about the patient's motives and may suggest the best course of action. Get the story in detail. Determine the level of lethality and the intent to die. What did the patient do? How long had the patient been thinking about it? What preparations were made? How was the attempt discovered? Was medical treatment required? Was the patient hospitalized?

Questions of lethality are of primary concern because, regardless of the seriousness of suicidal intent, patients who use lethal means are at higher risk for death. Patients who swallow a bottle of acetaminophen in a fit of pique, unaware of the potential for hepatic injury, are probably in greater danger through sheer recklessness than patients who swallow what they believe to be a lethal dose of 10 aspirins.

The seriousness of suicidal intent can be assessed in two ways. First, the physician can ask the patient directly: "Did you want to die? Did you expect to die?" Second, seriousness can be deduced from the details of the patient's behavior. Was the patient alone? If alone, was there a reasonable expectation of rapid discovery? Did the patient tell anyone before the event or call someone immediately after? Was the interest in self-destruction sustained long enough to make careful preparations, or was the attempt made on impulse, using only the means at hand?

A patient who studies the *Physicians' Desk Reference* for information about the adverse effects of drug overdose and who plans to be alone and undiscovered for hours after the ingestion is more serious about dying than a patient who swallows a few pills in the heat of an argument. The risk of a fatal suicide attempt in the future is directly proportional to the lethality of the means used and the degree to which the patient plans for and works to ensure the completion of the suicidal act. Patients who have recently survived a planned suicide attempt and are not yet fully recovered from an underlying psychiatric illness are at high risk of dying by their own hand in the near future.

Patients Who Acknowledge Suicidal Thoughts but Have Not Injured Themselves

- *An elderly widower mutters, as he is buttoning his shirt after a checkup, that he has been wrestling with the idea of joining his wife.*

- *A distraught parent calls to read the suicide note found in a teenager's notebook.*

- *A patient in the office requests a prescription refill and then tearfully confides having had thoughts of taking the whole bottle at once.*

- *After making a long list of complaints, a patient sighs, "Oh, I wish I were dead."*

- *A new patient with a chronic illness asks the physician's position on doctor-assisted suicide.*

- *A patient with depression acknowledges suicidal fantasies, but only when asked about them.*

Primary care physicians should treat any of these scenarios as they would complaints of chest pain: just as chest pain is a myocardial infarction until proven otherwise, suicidal thoughts imply lethal intent until proven otherwise. As with the assessment of past suicidal behavior, the assessment of a suicidal statement hinges on the seriousness of intent and the lethality and specificity of the plan. Most patients, when challenged about a vague suicidal statement, will offer a retraction: "Oh, I would never do that [to my family/because of my religion/because I'm a coward]." Such retractions are reassuring, especially if they are repeated.

Patients who do not retract suicidal thoughts or who hedge their retractions ("I have no intention of killing myself—today") require further assessment. Ask them what brought on the thoughts, how often they occur, and how difficult they are to shake. Do the thoughts include a plan? If so, what is it? Patients with a mild risk of suicide may have no plan at all, just a vague desire to escape, to be dead, or to become oblivious. Other patients may offer a plan in some detail: "I thought of [taking an overdose/buying a gun/jumping off a building]." Here, the physician should ask if the patient has thought about what drug to take, where to buy a gun, or which tall buildings have roof access? Such questions will not move the ambivalent patient closer to suicide. Patients at serious risk for a lethal attempt, in revealing their plans, offer the physician specific ways to intervene (e.g., by insisting that firearms be removed from the home or that a cache of old prescription drugs be destroyed).

The risk of suicidal behavior rises with the persistence of suicidal intent, the specificity of the plan, and the availability of means. Patients who retract their suicidal statement or whose thoughts on suicide have no specific content are at the lowest risk for self-injurious behavior. Patients who have a plan for committing suicide but who express firm personal prohibitions about the act are at somewhat higher risk. In an exacerbation of a depressive illness or in the midst of an alcohol binge, personal ethics (and such patients) may go out the window. More troubling are patients who have researched their plan, rehearsed it mentally, or taken preliminary steps to set it in motion. Most worrisome of all are patients who have survived a suicide attempt, however mild, but continue to express suicidal thoughts.

To estimate a patient's potential for suicide, the primary care physician should understand not only the degree of intent and the lethality and specificity of the plan, but also other aspects of the patient's mental state and behavior. Demographic profiles of suicide risk add something to the assessment of individual cases but are of less value than descriptions of how the patient has been thinking, feeling, and acting. Depressive disorders, as we have seen, put patients at increased risk for suicide. Severely depressed patients—especially those with low self-esteem and feelings of guilt—often express the belief that their family or the world would be better off without them. Among the signs of depression that predict suicide, hopelessness is the most powerful. Giving away possessions or writing a will may be an important clue to hopelessness, but it is by no means prerequisite to a serious attempt. A direct way to uncover feelings of hopelessness is to ask the patient: "How does the future look to you?"

Safety Considerations

Suicidal thinking constitutes an emergency when the patient cannot provide assurances of safety. A patient who cannot convincingly retract a suicidal statement, avow abstinence from suicidal behavior, or produce a foolproof plan of family monitoring should be referred to an emergency room for psychiatric evaluation—with or without the patient's agreement. If the patient is already hospitalized, the primary care physician should request a prompt psychiatric consultation.

Retracted Suicidal Statements

When patients make suicidal or nihilistic utterances and then take them back, the physician's decision to accept the retraction as an assurance of safety hinges on his or her level of comfort with the patient's sincerity and judgment. Patients who describe carefully elaborated plans or who have made preparations to act on them have invested so much effort toward suicide that momentary backpedaling in the office should raise suspicions of insincerity. Likewise, patients who have a history of impulsive behavior may in all sincerity deny suicidal intent for the moment but risk another flare-up at home. The physician might have a lower threshold for sending home a compliant patient with whom he or she has a longstanding relationship than a new patient or a patient with a track record of poor follow-through. Patients who own firearms can demonstrate their sincerity by arranging to remove them from the home. Refusal to do so casts doubt on the sincerity of the patient's retraction.

"Contracts" for Safety

The primary care physician can sometimes decide to send a patient with suicidal thinking home rather than to the emergency room if the patient has low intent, finds it possible to ignore the thoughts, and can be relied on to honor a promise not to act on any suicidal impulses. Patients who cannot give blanket assurances of this sort may at least be able to promise not to act until the next visit, which should be scheduled within a few days, depending on the particulars of the case. Having the patient write out and sign a statement for the medical record has the dual advantage of cementing the patient's resolve not to act on suicidal impulses and of documenting the physician's discussion with the patient about suicide. If there is any doubt about the patient's ability or willingness to honor this promise (past performance being a strong predictor), the patient should be referred for emergency psychiatric evaluation.

Family Monitoring

Well-informed families can provide lifesaving support. A patient who might otherwise require psychiatric hospitalization may go home with a spouse, parents, or children if the suicide risk is low and the family is aware of the danger and up to the task of keeping track of the patient's mental state and whereabouts. Patients thinking of suicide who refuse to allow family members to know of their condition place themselves and the physician in an intolerably risky position. A patient's reluctance to accept family support undermines a promise to abstain from suicidal behavior and should trigger consideration of an emergency psychiatric referral.

Psychiatric Referral Options

Emergency Referral. A patient deemed at high risk for suicide warrants hospitalization. If the patient already has a psychiatrist, the psychiatrist may admit the patient directly; if not, admission should be sought through an emergency room. Here are some pointers regarding emergency referral:

—Family members or an ambulance should take the patient to the emergency room. It is too risky to allow the patient to drive to an emergency room alone.

—Suicidal patients who refuse to go to an emergency room can be brought there by the police. The details of such involuntary evaluations vary from state to state, and physicians should have access to those appropriate for the jurisdiction in which they practice.

—Call ahead to inform the emergency room staff about the suicidal patient. Some patients, on arrival to the emergency room, will minimize the concerns of the referring physician.

Outpatient Psychiatric Evaluation. Patients with suicidal thoughts who are at low risk for suicidal behavior warrant referral for outpatient psychiatric care under some circumstances. Patients with significant impairment from a major depression or who have difficulty tolerating or responding to antidepressant treatment should be so referred. Patients with incorrigible substance abuse may require referral to a detoxification/rehabilitation program. Patients with fleeting or vague suicidal thoughts, when these thoughts seem related to a stressful situation, may respond to counseling, either with a nonphysician psychotherapist or with the primary care physician. Frequent, brief visits with the primary care physician to talk in concrete terms about the stresses that led to the suicidal thoughts may help a patient through a crisis. Patients at low risk whose suicidal thoughts do not abate in the context of substance abuse treatment or psychotherapy should be referred for psychiatric assessment, as should those whose psychological state is unclear or whose medical conditions are complicated.

When outpatient psychiatric evaluation is chosen, the primary care physician should be knowledgeable about the treatment setting to which the patient has been referred. How soon can the patient be seen? Do psychiatrists or psychologists perform evaluations, or must patients undergo a screening process by nurses or social workers before being referred to a psychiatrist? Can the primary care physician make the appointment, or must the patient call for one? Any added step between the patient and an evaluation by a specialist able to assess and treat the source of suicidal thinking is a chance for treatment to stumble and for suicidal thoughts to become suicidal behavior. Patients who are ambivalent about discussing suicidal thoughts with the primary care physician are unlikely to arrange a psychiatric evaluation on their own. Nonphysician intake counselors may be more likely to accept a patient's attempts to explain away symptoms and thus may fail to move the patient quickly toward needed antidepressant treatment. The prompt availability of psychiatric outpatient evaluation or the lack thereof should factor into the decision about whether to refer a suicidal patient to an emergency room.

Psychiatric Evaluation for Inpatients. Patients hospitalized for medical illness or surgical procedures are, by the fact of their confinement, under severe stress. Some of these patients may have major depression; many more are demoralized. In this situation, frightened by the body's dysfunction, taken from home, and deprived of supporting relationships, patients sometimes express a wish for death as an alternative to the suffering and uncertainty of illness. The evaluation of these statements is the same as when they are made in the physician's office.

It may be tempting for the primary care physician to request a psychiatric consultation as soon as the patient mentions a wish to die. Psychiatric consultation will be more valuable, if it is needed at all, after the primary care physician has done an assessment. Statements expressing a passive preference for death generally require only reassurance or clarification, perhaps in the form of a more detailed discussion of the treatment and prognosis of the illness that is distressing the patient. Suicidal statements more specific in content and lethal in implication, especially when associated with a psychiatric disorder, do warrant specialty consultation.

Primary Care for Patients with Suicidal Thoughts

In many cases, stable patients with fleeting suicidal thoughts who are at low risk for self-injury can be treated by their primary care physicians. Even when the physician requests psychiatric referral, he or she should see the patient in follow-up if the consultation is delayed for a week or more.

Antidepressant Therapy

As discussed in Chapter 2, patients with major depression should be started on antidepressant medication. It is essential for the primary care physician to keep in mind two risks inherent in treating the suicidal patient with major depression. First, many of the older generation of antidepressants (tricyclic antidepressants like amitriptyline hydrochloride, imipramine hydrochloride, nortriptyline hydrochloride, and doxepin hydrochloride) can be fatal in overdose. If there is a good reason for prescribing such a drug (e.g., prior response, inability to afford the newer drugs, formulary limitations), it is usually safe to prescribe a week's worth of medication at a time. At low starting doses, this quantity should not provide the means for a potentially fatal overdose. Most of the time it will be preferable to prescribe a selective serotonin reuptake inhibitor (SSRI), such as fluoxetine hydrochloride, paroxetine hydrochloride, or sertraline hydrochloride, which are extremely unlikely to have fatal consequences in overdose.

The second caveat in treating the depressed patient with suicidal thoughts is that the early weeks of treatment can be the most dangerous for self-injury. Full antidepressant response can take six to eight weeks. Patients with suicidal ideas in the context of depressive lethargy and inertia may exhibit a more active drive toward suicide in the early phases of antidepressant treatment, when physical energy and activity increase but the mood remains low. It is essential for the primary care physician to follow the patient closely, no less frequently than once a week, in the early weeks of antidepressant treatment. Patients and family members should be made aware of avenues for the immediate availability of help if the patient's depression should worsen between visits or if the patient becomes agitated. If there is doubt about the patient's safety between visits, inpatient treatment is probably warranted.

Psychological Support

Suicidal thoughts sometimes emerge without signs of major depression in patients encountering difficult situations. By the first follow-up visit after these thoughts have been discussed, the physician may find the patient more hopeful and perhaps dismissive of the suicidal remarks previously made. If, on reevaluation, it appears to the physician and family that the patient does not have a depressive disorder, the problem may be over. These patients may or may not benefit from counseling to learn how to avoid another crisis.

Patients with persistent suicidal thoughts require repeated monitoring to establish their safety. Monitoring itself can be felt as supportive; patients are assured that the physician, at least, cares whether they live or die. After asking how the patient is feeling, the physician can ask: "You told me last time we spoke that you were having thoughts of ending your life. I wonder whether those thoughts are still with you?" Physicians should not only lend a sympathetic ear to the patient's complaints, but also challenge, gently but persistently, the patient's nihilistic statements. Patients who have begun to rationalize suicide, who state, for example, that their families would be better off without them, may be reminded that suicide is always an indelibly horrible experience for those left behind.

Summary

Suicide is a leading cause of premature death and is associated with depression, alcoholism, and other common psychiatric and medical disorders. The primary care physician should screen for depressed mood both patients with obvious emotional disturbance or psychiatric illness and patients facing situations of loss or distress. When depression is present, a discussion about suicidal thoughts should follow. When patients express suicidal thoughts, the primary care physician's immediate task is to ensure safety, by referral to an emergency room if necessary. Safety can be assessed by understanding the seriousness of the patient's suicidal intent and the specificity and lethality of any suicidal plans. The availability of firearms raises the risk of death by suicide significantly. Among the additional factors to consider in deciding on the most appropriate course of treatment are the patient's history of past suicidal behavior, the presence or absence of a psychiatric disorder, and the availability of social support and specialized treatment.

REFERENCES

Anderson, Robert N.; Kolchanek, Kenneth D.; and Murphy, Sherry L. Report of Final Mortality Statistics, 1995. *Monthly Vital Statistics Report* 45 (1997): Supplement 2.

Harris, E. Clare, and Barraclough, Brian M. Suicide as an Outcome for Medical Disorders. *Medicine* 73 (1994): 281–296.

Hendin, Herbert. Suicide, Assisted Suicide, and Medical Illness. *Journal of Clinical Psychiatry* 60, suppl. 2 (1999): 46–50.

Inskip, Hazel M.; Harris, E. Clare; and Barraclough, Brian. Lifetime Risk of Suicide for Affective Disorder, Alcoholism and Schizophrenia. *British Journal of Psychiatry* 172 (1998): 35–37.

Isometsä, Erkki T., and Lönnqvist, Juoko K. Suicide Attempts Preceding Completed Suicide. *British Journal of Psychiatry* 173 (1998): 531–535.

Jamison, Kay R. *Night Falls Fast: Understanding Suicide.* New York: Alfred Knopf, 1999.

Pirkis, Jane, and Burgess, Philip. Suicide and Recency of Health Care Contacts: A Systematic Review. *British Journal of Psychiatry* 173 (1998): 462–474.

Stoff, David M., and Mann, J. John, editors. The Neurobiology of Suicide: From the Bench to the Clinic. *Annals of the New York Academy of Sciences* 836 (1997).

SEVEN

Dependence on Alcohol or Drugs

Alan J. Romanoski, M.D., M.P.H.

The most common diagnosable psychiatric disorders encountered in primary care are those involving the self-administration of psychoactive substances. Psychoactive substances have two characteristics: (1) they affect the way one feels, thinks, or acts; and (2) their repeated use can become self-sustaining. A psychoactive substance use disorder is a persistent pattern of behavior whose focus is on acquiring and using such drugs.

Nearly 25 percent of adults either drink alcoholic beverages in this way or are vulnerable to doing so, and the analogous rate for tobacco smoking approximates 35 percent. In many major U.S. cities, 10 percent of adults use heroin daily, with the rate for cocaine not far behind. Suburban and rural areas, once thought relatively insulated from these latter problems, are now witnessing exponential increases in illicit drug use. Among homeless individuals and those who are infected with human immunodeficiency virus (HIV), substance use disorders are the rule rather than the exception.

Although substance use disorders are mostly self-inflicted, they can be initiated or sustained through the well-intentioned treatment of a variety of common complaints (e.g., anxiety, headaches, insomnia, chronic pain). For most front-line practitioners, few days go by without repeated requests for more or stronger psychoactive medications. Once a substance use disorder has become established, it brings its own cargo of medical and psychiatric problems.

Properties of Psychoactive Drugs

It has long been common to ascribe substance use disorders to weakness of the patient's will, to characterologic flaws, or to temperamental vulnerabilities. To adopt this posture is, however, to ignore the fact that psychoactive drugs all have two pharmacologic properties that distinguish them from other agents, are responsible for their virulence, and underlie the rationale for their close regulation by governmental agencies: their *abuse liability* and their *withdrawal potential.* Repeated exposure to such substances, whether via experimentation or prescription, can change brain function in fundamental and long-lasting ways that are difficult to overcome once established.

Abuse Liability

Abuse liability refers to the strength of an agent's self-reinforcing properties—its intrinsic effects that increase the likelihood that it will be taken again. Psychoactive substances differ from one another in the relative strength of their abuse liability. Cocaine is the standard against which the abuse liability of other agents is measured: laboratory animals will work harder for cocaine than for other agents and may die of starvation when given the choice of cocaine versus food, even if the cocaine is made extremely difficult to obtain. Amphetamine, other stimulants, and cannabis have high abuse liabilities compared to alcohol and nicotine, while those for opioids and barbiturates are less strong. Benzodiazepines tend to have the lowest abuse liabilities of common psychoactive drugs.

An agent's abuse liability can be markedly modified by its preparation and mode of administration, both of which determine the speed and concentration with which it reaches the brain. For example, the absorption of intranasal cocaine is aided by the high vascularity of the nasal mucosa but limited by the mucosa's small surface area and by the drug's own vasoconstrictive properties. When cocaine is smoked, it can be delivered to the bloodstream in much larger amounts, and when it is prepared as "crack" (which vaporizes at a lower temperature), it can be inhaled with less discomfort, so even more can be delivered. By contrast, the range of alcohol's abuse liability is narrowed by inherent limitations in the way it can be taken (i.e., in beverage form).

Withdrawal Potential

The *withdrawal potential* of an agent refers to the relative ease with which reduction in its persistent use can provoke a stereotypic cluster of symptoms and signs—an abstinence syndrome. Abstinence syndromes can occur even without evidence of physiologic tolerance (i.e., without the need for increasing doses to achieve the same effect). Thus, for example, patients who have taken maintenance doses of benzodiazepines for months to years without having acquired physiologic tolerance often experience an abstinence syndrome with abrupt reduction in dose.

The term *withdrawal* is sometimes restricted to observable physiologic derangements (e.g., signs of autonomic overactivity) and not applied to a variety of unpleasant subjective states that are relieved by further use of the drug. This limitation is inappropriate, for phenomena such as hallucinations and cravings for the substance in question are regular parts of abstinence syndromes. Withdrawal symptoms and signs for specific agents are shown in Table 7.1.

Among psychoactive drugs, opioids generally have the highest withdrawal potential. Opioid-naive patients with high analgesic requirements, such as those with severe pain due to burns, often experience significant withdrawal after only weeks of use in doses required for adequate pain relief. Barbiturate users can develop withdrawal symptoms in weeks to months, and benzodiazepine users in months to years. Patients taking second-generation benzodiazepines such as alprazolam and clonazepam seem to develop abstinence syndromes more quickly and of greater severity than those using first-generation agents such as diazepam. Compared to these drugs, the withdrawal potentials of nicotine and alcohol are moderate, and those of cocaine and cannabis are modest.

Given an agent's withdrawal potential, the risk of developing a withdrawal syndrome is largely a function of the quantity, frequency, and persistence of use. Individuals with a high degree of tolerance are more likely

Table 7.1. Abstinence Syndromes for Psychoactive Agents

Opioids
  Intense craving for opioids
  Pulse or blood pressure elevation, or both
  Mild temperature elevation
  Dilated pupils
  Piloerection, or recurrent chills and/or sweats
  Lacrimation, rhinorrhea, or sneezing
  Abdominal cramps, nausea, vomiting,
    diarrhea
  Muscle aches and cramps
  Restlessness, psychomotor agitation
  Anxiety or other affective distress
  Insomnia
  Malaise
Benzodiazepines, sedatives, hypnotics
  Pulse or blood pressure elevation, or both
  Postural hypotension
  Mild temperature elevation
  Sweating
  Tremulousness, fasciculations
  Migratory pains and paresthesias
  Nausea, vomiting
  Headache
  Tinnitus
  Restlessness, psychomotor agitation
  Anxiety or other affective distress
  Hypervigilance (e.g., hyperacusis,
    startle response)
  Insomnia
  Malaise, weakness
  Paranoid ideation
  Depersonalization, derealization
  Transient visual, tactile, or auditory
    hallucinations or illusions
  Major withdrawal: delirium, generalized
    seizures, hallucinosis
Alcohol
  Pulse or blood pressure elevation, or both
  Postural hypotension
  Mild temperature elevation
  Sweating
  Tremulousness, fasciculations
  Nausea, vomiting
  Facial edema
  Headache
  Restlessness, psychomotor agitation
  Anxiety or other affective distress
  Insomnia
  Malaise, weakness
  Transient visual, tactile, or auditory
    hallucinations or illusions
  Major withdrawal: delirium, generalized
    seizures, hallucinosis

Nicotine
  Craving for nicotine
  Increased appetite
  Coughing
  Restlessness, psychomotor agitation
  Irritability
  Anxiety or other affective distress
  Insomnia
  Malaise, weakness
Cocaine
  Intense craving for cocaine
  Slowed pulse
  Headaches
  Restlessness, psychomotor agitation
  Irritability, anger
  Anxiety
  Depression, suicidal ideation
  Drowsiness, hypersomnia, followed by
    insomnia
  Bizarre or unpleasant dreams
  Increased appetite, increased food
    consumption, weight gain
  Lethargy, fatigue, exhaustion
Stimulants other than cocaine
  Craving for drug
  Psychomotor retardation, followed by
    agitation
  Hypersomnia, followed by insomnia
  Bizarre or unpleasant dreams
  Increased appetite
  Lethargy, fatigue
Cannabinoids
  Various symptoms (e.g., craving,
    irritability) after prolonged high-dose
    use have been described, but no
    stereotyped syndrome has been
    validated.
Hallucinogens
  None

to experience withdrawal symptoms, but the converse is not necessarily true. A withdrawal syndrome may begin while someone is still using a psychoactive substance if use has declined from a previously established level. As will be discussed below, the most accurate predictor of withdrawal symptoms in the future is a withdrawal syndrome in the past.

The abuse liability of an agent sustains its use when the user likes its effect so much that it becomes increasingly difficult to resist. The withdrawal potential of an agent sustains its use when the user finds that more must be taken purely to relieve or avoid its abstinence syndrome.

The Concepts of Dependence, Abuse, and Harmful Use

Traditionally, substance use disorders have been dichotomized into the categories of "dependence" and nondependent "abuse." Distinctions were drawn between psychological and physiologic dependence: the former connoting an emotional need or behavioral habit of drug taking; the latter, a physical state characterized by the phenomena of tolerance and physiologic withdrawal. On the basis of such logic, it was widely held until the last decade that cocaine and cannabis could not provoke "true" dependence because abstinence did not produce observable physiologic withdrawal. Such a restricted definition is misleading. The term *dependence* is better understood as the use of a psychoactive substance that has become an irreplaceable part of daily life, even if physiologic withdrawal has not occurred.

The concept of drug abuse has also proven problematic. Because people take intoxicants to become intoxicated, stimulants to become stimulated, and mood-altering drugs to alter their moods, they can reject the term *abuse* to describe their behavior. What they are doing, they say, is taking the agent for its intended purpose, often in a "recreational" manner. One way to avoid arguments with patients about whether or not they are drug abusers is to use the term *harmful use*—persistent use despite demonstrably adverse physical, social, or psychological consequences.

Elements of Dependence Syndromes

Dependence syndromes comprise the following elements, all of which tend to co-vary:

—Narrowed pattern of use
—Increased importance of continued use
—Acquisition of increased tolerance
—Attempted prevention of withdrawal symptoms
—Awareness of a compulsion to use
—Impaired control over use
—Reinstatement of the full syndrome after abstinence

A Narrowed Pattern of Use

Patients who once varied their choice of agent and the amount, manner, and timing of its use in accordance with social circumstances begin to use the same agent in the same amount prepared in the same way and at the same time, regardless of whether they are alone or with others and whether it is a weekday or a weekend.

The Increased Importance of Continued Use

Patients escalate their use of the drug despite the fact that its once-perceived benefits come to be outweighed by its deleterious effects. Time spent acquiring, using, and recovering from the drug progressively replaces time devoted to activities formerly given higher priorities (e.g., nurturing relationships, maintaining one's livelihood). Ever-worsening consequences, including life-threatening illness, fail to deter further use.

The Acquisition of Increased Tolerance

In the development of a dependence syndrome, amounts of a drug once sufficient to produce a certain effect now fail to do so. Patients who were previously tolerant to large quantities of a drug will become less so if they sustain brain or hepatic injury.

Tolerance to one class of drugs often provokes but does not invariably predict cross-tolerance to another. Patients with a high tolerance to alcohol, for example, readily develop similar tolerance to benzodiazepines, barbiturates, and anesthetic agents. A relationship exists between alcohol and opioids such that acetaldehyde, alcohol's first metabolite, has been linked to increased production of endogenous opiates in the brain, which may explain the increased affinity for opioids observed among alcoholic persons and the frequency with which chronic pain patients develop alcoholism. Not all cross-tolerance is complete, however—a fact with important implications for the treatment of withdrawal states.

The Attempted Prevention of Withdrawal Symptoms

Patients who experience abstinence syndromes quickly learn that "replacement therapy," with either the offending agent or a pharmacologic substitute, provides prompt—if temporary—relief. Many such patients get caught in a vicious cycle of increasing use and worsening withdrawal, develop a keen sense of their own dose-response curves, and begin to use the drug as prophylaxis against impending withdrawal. They may attempt to obtain multiple prescriptions when they are dependent on a medication and may hide their drugs or alcohol to ensure always having a supply at hand. Many patients dependent on alcohol will admit to "predrinking"—consuming alcohol before entering situations in which access to it may be limited.

The Awareness of a Compulsion to Use

The repeated urge to use can be experienced as a craving, which is readily acknowledged by most cocaine and heroin addicts. Patients dependent on alcohol may deny craving when asked about it directly but usually admit to a "taste" for beer that leads them to consume five or more in a single sitting. Patients often admit to self-imposed measures to resist further use (e.g., keeping busy, not permitting alcohol in the home, restricting access to ready cash for the purchase of drugs).

Impaired Control over Use

Patients who intend to take only one or two drinks or doses of drug increasingly find that they end up taking a much larger amount for a much longer period than intended. Each dose increases the desire for another. For example, consumption of a single drink often leads to drinking to intoxication, if not an alcoholic "blackout." Such binges are terminated by sickness, functional incapacity, or social adversity rather than by satiety.

Reinstatement of the Full Dependence Syndrome after Abstinence

Abstinence does not extinguish dependence. This is the cardinal feature of the dependence syndrome. No matter how long they have been drug-free, most dependent patients who resume drug use reacquire the dependence syndrome within days to weeks. For example, alcoholic patients who relapse after months of incarceration—and enforced abstinence—can develop full-blown alcohol withdrawal after bingeing for only 24–48 hours.

The mechanism for this reinstatement phenomenon seems to be learning through neural memory, habituation, and behavioral conditioning. Establishment of a dependence syndrome results from a complex, integrated interaction of central nervous system processes. In this way it is not unlike learning to ride a bicycle (another complex, integrated task): once one learns, one never forgets, no matter how long one is out of the saddle.

Risk Factors

Psychoactive substance use disorders are best understood by using the infectious disease model of interactions among pathogenic agents (psychoactive substances), hosts (users), and environmental factors. The complementary roles of an agent's abuse liability and its withdrawal potential have been previously described. Many individuals can rapidly become dependent on cocaine or stimulants even in the absence of observable physical withdrawal, while others can become dependent on benzodiazepines despite their relatively low abuse liability.

Although accurate phenotyping of an "addictive personality" has proved elusive, many dispositional, genetic, and environmental factors render some users more vulnerable to substance use disorders. If the primary care physician can identify those patients at risk for the development of dependence, he or she can perhaps prevent users from becoming regular users, regular users from becoming harmful ones, and harmful users from becoming dependent.

For unknown reasons, the state induced by psychoactive substances is more intrinsically rewarding to some persons than to others. The only way to find out is to take a careful history: to ask about use of each class of drug and its effects. For example, stimulants cause some patients to feel energized or euphoric but others to feel unpleasantly excited or jittery.

For a variety of cultural, social, and genetic reasons, men are more likely than women to develop substance use disorders. For example, consuming alcohol is commonly held to be more compatible with masculinity than femininity, drinking to intoxication has become an adolescent male "rite of passage" in colleges and other settings, and sex differences in the amount and activity of alcohol dehydrogenase enable males to tolerate higher doses of alcohol without intoxication. Such factors increase the likelihood that males will get more repeated exposures to alcohol than will females.

A positive family history of any substance use disorder suggests strong genetic or environmental loading for the development of dependence. Patients with a personal history of drug use and a current psychiatric disorder are at increased risk; the more severe the psychopathology, the higher the risk. Environmental factors also play a role in the development of dependence, over and above such obvious influences as the availability, accessibility, and affordability of psychoactive substances and the social acceptance or stigmatization of their use. For example, jobs in the hotel and restaurant trades, public relations, advertising, and entertainment, as well as unskilled, seasonal, and day labor, are associated with increased risk.

In general, the greater the psychosocial burden of one who has become a regular user of an agent, the greater the likelihood of developing dependency. For example, persons who drink regularly are much more likely to become alcohol-dependent on becoming widowed, divorced, retired, or disabled.

Finally, a change in the preparation or route of administration of an agent can be highly predictive of dependence. Persons who convert from using cocaine or heroin intranasally to smoking it are likely to become dependent in weeks to months, and those who convert from smoking to intravenous use are likely to become dependent in days to weeks.

Diagnosis

Psychoactive substance use disorders are most accurately diagnosed by history. The "CAGE-B" questionnaire (Table 7.2), which has been adapted from the CAGE to include all classes of psychoactive drugs rather than alcohol alone, can be used to elicit such a history. The physician should always ask other informants for their observations or concerns about a patient's alcohol and drug use. The physician should ask some patients for whom he or she prescribes controlled substances for permission to contact their pharmacy and other physicians to make sure that multiple prescriptions are not being written. The physician should assume that any patient who regularly inhales, smokes, or injects any agent has a dependency syndrome until proven otherwise.

Not all patients are readily forthcoming with history or permit contact with other informants. Thus, the physician should remember that certain signs on the physical examination can indicate psychoactive substance use. Multiple tattoos or body piercings may reflect a disregard for societal norms, including those that limit drug taking. Facial or digital edema, cigarette-stained fingers, palmar erythema, and spider nevi suggest alcohol dependence, and any odor of beverage alcohol is more than a little suggestive of the same. Tremor, tachycardia, elevated blood pressure, and dilated pupils may indicate repeated ingestion of alcohol, barbiturates, benzodiazepines, or other sedatives. Nasal septal necrosis suggests repeated cocaine use, while dilated pupils and multiple scars and keloids on the extremities suggest intravenous drug use, usually heroin or cocaine. Miosis, decreased bowel sounds, flaccid muscles, and urinary retention can be due to opioids.

Laboratory studies may also be helpful in the diagnosis of psychoactive substance use disorders. Thus, thrombocytopenia, high mean corpuscular volume, and elevations of serum uric acid, aspartate aminotransferase, and gamma glutamyltransferase suggest heavy drinking. Liver function studies, especially alkaline phosphatase, are often elevated in chronic opioid users.

Table 7.2. CAGE-B

C: Have you felt the need to Cut down on your drug/alcohol use?
A: Do people Annoy you by commenting on your drug/alcohol use?
G: Have you ever felt Guilty about your drug/alcohol use?
E: Have you ever needed an Eye opener or had to use drugs/alcohol daily just to feel normal?

B: Have you ever had two or more Blackouts so that you couldn't remember what you did?

Affirmative responses to **B** or to two or more **CAGE** questions indicate positive screening for substance use disorder.

Handheld devices that screen for ethanol in expired air can be used to discern whether a patient's breath smells of alcohol or something else.

Any suspicion of drug use should be followed by a urine toxicology screen. Cocaine and its metabolites can persist in the urine for 48–96 hours, especially after an episode of heavy use. Opioids, with the exception of methadone, clear more quickly. Hydrocodone is often undetectable in the urine unless it has been used in high doses. Quinine and quinidine, which are used to dilute cocaine and heroin, often remain in the urine for several days to a week.

Phenobarbital can be detected in the urine for well over a week, while shorter-acting barbiturates such as butalbital disappear much more rapidly. Benzodiazepines with long half-lives (e.g., diazepam, chlordiazepoxide hydrochloride, and clonazepam) can persist for well over a week, especially in elderly patients. Shorter-acting benzodiazepines (e.g., alprazolam, triazolam) often escape detection in the urine except when used in large doses.

Alcohols, including isopropyl, can be detected and quantified in a blood volatile screen. Other drugs—either suspected or initially detected in the urine—can also be quantified in the blood.

Discussing the Diagnosis with the Patient

The primary care physician should tell patients who use drugs in a harmful way but do not have a dependence syndrome of the risks they are running. If a dependence syndrome is present, the physician should first explain exactly what that diagnosis means (i.e., that a drug has become an essential part of the patient's daily life and is endangering his or her health, relationships, and employment). The physician should then provide evidence for the diagnosis based on the history, examination, and laboratory findings. In general, patients are more likely to accept the diagnosis when it is linked to withdrawal symptoms (e.g., morning "shakes") or abnormal laboratory findings than when it is linked to an automobile accident, a poor job evaluation, or family friction.

The term *denial* refers to a patient's refusal to acknowledge the extent or consequences of his or her drug use. Denial can range from a genuine lack of enlightenment, to embarrassed minimizing, to equivocation, to outright lying. Telling patients that they "abuse" alcohol or drugs or are failing in their role performance may only make them incredulous, defensive, or angry. It is far more persuasive to explain to them how rare it is for someone to have their symptoms (e.g., blackouts), laboratory findings, and behaviors (e.g., drinking on awakening) *without* having a substance use disorder. Patients who insist that laboratory results are erroneous should be invited to have them repeated. Denial is best countered with facts, logic, and the stated desire to come to a mutual understanding of what otherwise would be a mysterious association of phenomena.

Patients with dependence syndromes may be so oblivious to the importance of their drug-seeking behavior that they give only lip service to the knowledge that continued use may render irreversible the physical, psychological, or social harm they have already sustained. In such cases, the physician should consider a formal *intervention*—a confrontation by family or friends that generates a crisis whose favorable resolution can be achieved only by the patient's acceptance of treatment. Interventions should be carried out only by a clinical addictions counselor (CAC) or a psychiatrist, psychologist, nurse, or social worker with experience and expertise in this area.

Labeling psychoactive substance use disorders as diseases has advantages: it acknowledges that successful treatment requires more than sheer will, it permits a person to assume the patient role less shamefully, and it legitimizes resource allocation for treatment and prevention. Such labeling also has a major disadvantage: it implies diminished accountability of patients for their behavior, its consequences, and the outcome of treatment. Although physicians can help patients with dependence syndromes, the patients must do most of the work. For this reason, I do not think patients with psychoactive substance use disorders should be told they have a disease.

Treatment

No treatment uniformly applied to all patients with any alcohol or drug use disorder has ever been shown to be more effective than any other. Treatment must therefore address specific interactions among the offending drug, the patient's vulnerabilities, and the environment. All treatments can be thought of as having four stages: (1) closure on a concrete plan, (2) implementation of the plan, (3) preventive maintenance, and (4) relapse management. Regardless of the substance involved, all treatment plans have three essential steps: (1) stopping the drug-taking behavior and detoxifying the patient, (2) identifying and neutralizing factors that sustain drug-taking behavior, and (3) establishing a program to extinguish the habitual aspects of the behavior.

Closure on a Plan

Once physician and patient have agreed on the diagnosis, they should immediately close on a coherent, stepwise treatment plan. At every stage of treatment, there should be agreement on a backup plan (e.g., inpatient detoxification) if the first plan (e.g., outpatient detoxification) fails. Involvement of immediate family members, close friends, or both is important not only at this point, but also at every treatment stage.

The remainder of this chapter will focus on the treatment of alcohol, opioid, cocaine, and sedative use disorders. Smoking cessation programs and the treatment of stimulant, cannabis, and volatile solvent use disorders are beyond its scope.

Implementation of the Plan

Patients likely to experience withdrawal symptoms require detoxification. Past withdrawal symptoms are the best predictor of those in the future, and future withdrawal syndromes should be anticipated to be more severe than those of the past.

Many patients will seek detoxification simply to gain temporary relief from their withdrawal misery, but not every patient should necessarily be detoxified simply because of an expressed desire to do so. Any patient who has never undergone medical detoxification should be given the opportunity as quickly as possible, as should anyone active in treatment who relapses. Medical detoxification should always be undertaken whenever a patient's alcohol or drug use significantly compromises the treatment of any other disorder (e.g., epilepsy, diabetes, cardiovascular dysfunction, anxiety and depressive disorders). Otherwise, detoxification should be undertaken only when part of a broader, mutually agreed-upon, long-range treatment strategy in order to deter poorly motivated patients from employing "revolving door" detoxification as a stopgap measure (e.g., when their drug supply has been temporarily interrupted). A bit of clinical skepticism should be exercised with kindness.

Key to any detoxification is *quarantine*: sequestering of patients (hosts) from environments in which psychoactive substances (agents) are available.

There are nearly as many detoxification protocols as there are institutions, and no single one will prove right for most patients. With this caveat, suggested strategies follow.

Alcohol. A history of major withdrawal phenomena (e.g., delirium tremens, acute withdrawal hallucinosis, seizures) calls for inpatient detoxification. Fever or significant medical comorbidity (such as pneumonia or systemic infection, liver or other active gastrointestinal disease, a history of cardiac dysfunction, malnourishment, and recent trauma) is also an indication for inpatient detoxification. Patients with psychiatric disorders (such as major depression, mania, panic disorder, and schizophrenia) or who are using multiple psychoactive drugs are best detoxified on inpatient psychiatric units. Patients with histories of major alcohol withdrawal but who are otherwise healthy can sometimes be safely detoxified in residential treatment facilities that have 24-hour medical supervision. Detoxification in such facilities is indicated for patients who have failed outpatient detoxification, who have poor social supports, or who have a limited grasp of the seriousness of their condition.

Many patients can be successfully detoxified by the primary care physician on an outpatient basis, but only if the patient and physician are prepared to see each other briefly in the office on *at least* an every-other-day basis *and* if there is a responsible person who can provide 24-hour supervision (which includes accompanying the patient to appointments). This treatment supervisor should be present when the patient is given initial instructions and should have at least telephone access to the physician or a medical treatment facility (or both) on a 24-hour basis.

Outpatient detoxification should be attempted only once and only after the results of baseline laboratory studies, toxicology screens, and a complete physical examination are in hand. At each office visit, disulfiram should be given under supervision (see under "Preventive Maintenance," below), but only after patients have had a negative test for alcohol in their expired air. Patients should also be encouraged to attend Alcoholics Anonymous or other group treatment meetings on a daily basis.

Intermediate- and long-acting benzodiazepines such as lorazepam, oxazepam, diazepam, and chlordiazepoxide hydrochloride are the drugs of choice for pharmacologic detoxification because of the wide therapeutic window between doses that yield benefit and those that cause toxicity. The choice of benzodiazepine depends on the patient's age and hepatic function and on the environment in which detoxification will take place. Chlordiazepoxide hydrochloride has an average half-life of 24–48 hours but a much longer one in elderly patients and those with impaired hepatic function. It is the drug of choice for patients who are young and otherwise healthy and who will be relatively sparsely supervised. Diazepam has a half-life of about 24 hours and poses fewer hepatic- or age-related constraints. Oxazepam's half-life is 8–12 hours, making it the drug of choice for patients who are elderly or have compromised hepatic function. Lorazepam has a 12–18-hour half-life.

The acute onset of action of 25 mg of chlordiazepoxide hydrochloride is roughly equivalent to that of 5 mg of diazepam, 15 mg of oxazepam, and 1 mg of lorazepam. Due to differences in half-lives, giving a single 10-mg dose of diazepam is roughly equivalent to giving 30 mg of oxazepam, followed by 15 mg eight hours later, followed by 7.5 mg eight hours after that, and to giving 2 mg of lorazepam, followed by 1 mg 12 hours later.

For outpatient detoxification, it is recommended that the physician prescribe an initial supply of 10 or 15 pills of 25-mg chlordiazepoxide hydrochloride, 5-mg diazepam, 15-mg oxazepam, or 1-mg lorazepam. The patient should be instructed to take one tablet every hour until calm. An additional pill (i.e., two) should be taken every hour for the following parameters: pulse greater than 90, nervousness, or tremulousness. If, after 24 hours, the patient has taken more than eight pills, one should conclude that detoxification cannot be safely done in an outpatient setting.

If the patient has taken eight or fewer tablets the first day, the dosage should be subsequently tapered to discontinuation. Benzodiazepines may be tapered according to the following schedules: diazepam: days to taper = age rounded to the nearest decade/10; oxazepam/lorazepam: days to taper = (age rounded to the nearest decade + 20)/10. Thus, a healthy 24-year-old could be detoxified safely with diazepam in two days (20/10 = 2) or with oxazepam or lorazepam in four days ((20 + 20)/10 = 4). The last pill each day should be taken at bedtime. A fixed tapering schedule often proves impractical for chlordiazepoxide hydrochloride because of the long half-life of its metabolites, so after the first day, one pill should be taken on a prn basis every two hours only for the withdrawal parameters in the paragraph above. With a chlordiazepoxide hydrochloride taper, one pill should be taken at bedtime at the end of each day that a prn pill is taken, but none should be given at bedtime if no pill is taken during the day. If, in the course of tapering a benzodiazepine, the patient becomes somnolent or shows signs of intoxication, the dose should be reduced. For this reason, the physician should see the patient, together with the person providing supervision and counting pills, on at least an every-other-day basis.

As physiologic withdrawal is a potent sustaining factor for continued alcohol use, some have thought that relapse could be prevented with low-dose maintenance benzodiazepine therapy. However, many studies have shown that the longer patients are maintained on benzodiazepines, the greater the likelihood of relapse. Thus, maintenance benzodiazepines or those with exceedingly long half-lives (e.g., clonazepam) should not be used. Detoxification should be completed as quickly as possible, making the intermediate-acting benzodiazepines more desirable than the long-acting ones.

Some adjunctive agents should be used empirically at the start of medical detoxification. Three doses of magnesium oxide, 400 mg po q8h, can be given to help prevent seizures and hypomagnesemia. Thiamine hydrochloride, 100 mg po qd, should also be started and continued indefinitely. However, employment of other adjunctive agents (e.g., propranolol hydrochloride for tremulousness and tachycardia, phenytoin or carbamazepine to prevent seizures) should be avoided, as they raise the risk of delirium and can otherwise complicate treatment. Anticonvulsants have no role in preventing alcohol withdrawal seizures, except for patients with preexisting seizure disorders.

If anything goes awry with outpatient detoxification, the patient should immediately be admitted to a hospital or residential treatment facility with 24-hour medical supervision.

Cocaine. Cocaine withdrawal is characterized by intense drug cravings and the precipitous onset of depression that is often indistinguishable from major depression. This depressive syndrome usually subsides within days but can persist from weeks to months. It carries a high mortality from suicide rather than from physiologic perturbations. Cocaine users are 40–60 times more likely to attempt suicide than nonusers. Patients with suicidal ideation or a history of suicide attempts should be detoxified on an inpatient psychiatric unit. Otherwise, patients can be treated at home under 24-hour supervision by a responsible designee.

Cocaine withdrawal cravings and depression often respond quickly to tricyclic antidepressants. Desipramine hydrochloride is the agent most commonly used because it has relatively few anticholinergic side effects, but any tricyclic antidepressant will do. Desipramine hydrochloride should be started at 50 mg po qhs and increased to 300 mg po qhs, if necessary. Blood levels should be monitored, with 150–300 ng/ml considered the therapeutic range. Bupropion hydrochloride is an effective alternative for patients who cannot tolerate tricyclic antidepressants. The immediate-release form of the drug should be started at 75 mg qd and increased, if necessary, to 100 mg tid. (See Chapter 2 for a more detailed discussion of antidepressant dosing.) Patients undergoing outpatient detoxification should attend Narcotics Anonymous meetings (see below) or other drug treatment group meetings on a daily basis.

Opioids. The withdrawal potential of opioids is extremely high, and patients can experience severe physiologic withdrawal after only weeks of taking such drugs. Repeated use to avoid withdrawal is the most potent reinforcer of opioid dependence. Despite these considerations, outpatient detoxification can be attempted, though with the same caveats as for detoxification from alcohol.

Although withdrawal phenomena appear 8–12 hours after the cessation of opioid use, peak intensity is not reached until 48–72 hours, and acute symptoms can persist for four or five more days. For this reason, most conventional three-day inpatient detoxification protocols are, in and of themselves, unsuccessful in preventing relapse by patients who continue to experience withdrawal symptoms after they leave. Further detoxification on an outpatient basis is therefore required.

Patients who are dependent on heroin can be detoxified with methadone or buprenorphine hydrochloride. Methadone provides ideal substitution therapy for heroin detoxification because of its minimal euphoriant effects and 24-hour half-life. When methadone is used for detoxification, federal law mandates that it can be prescribed for only a single three-day period. As the lives of heroin addicts have become focused on drug-seeking activity that is outside the law, physicians should try to evaluate the patient's trustworthiness before giving him or her a methadone prescription. The starting dose of methadone should be 10 mg every hour until withdrawal symptoms have abated or until three doses have been given; the dose should then be tapered by 10 mg a day. In this way, a course of methadone, which should be followed by additional measures described below, can be completed in three days. If the taper is poorly tolerated, the physician should consider switching to buprenorphine hydrochloride (see below). If more than 30 mg of methadone is required for relief of symptoms, the patient should have inpatient or medically supervised residential detoxification.

Buprenorphine hydrochloride, an opioid agonist-antagonist, can be used either at the start of heroin detoxification or after a three-day methadone taper. It has a rapid onset of action and a half-life of 6–12 hours. Although buprenorphine hydrochloride is an effective medication, there are three complications to its use: (1) physicians must have approval from the Drug Enforcement Administration (DEA) to prescribe it for outpatient detoxification, (2) it is given intramuscularly, and (3) it can be administered only by appropriately licensed medical personnel. On weekends, methadone can be substituted for buprenorphine hydrochloride with patients who are compliant.

The initial dose of buprenorphine hydrochloride is 0.15 mg im, and it is repeated every hour until withdrawal symptoms abate or four doses have been given. The total dose used is given the next day on a bid basis (half the dose in each injection) and is subsequently tapered by 12.5–25 percent per day, so the medication is discontinued after 4–7 days. If, on the first day of treatment, four 0.15-mg doses do not significantly alleviate withdrawal symptoms, inpatient or residential detoxification is indicated.

Morphine-dependent patients are best detoxified using sustained-release morphine sulfate preparations. Similarly, patients dependent on oxycodone-containing compounds should be detoxified using sustained-release oxycodone hydrochloride preparations. To get started, calculate the amount of morphine sulfate or oxycodone hydrochloride the patient is currently taking per day. This amount will equal the total daily dose of sustained-release preparation to be taken, first on a q8h basis for 36–48 hours and then on a q12h basis with tapering to discontinuation over a week or two. For example, a patient taking 10 mg of oxycodone hydrochloride every four hours would have a total daily dose of 60 mg. Sustained-release oxycodone hydrochloride would then be given at 20 mg q8h for three doses, followed by 30 mg q12h for two doses, after which the taper to discontinuation on a q12h schedule should begin. Near the end of the taper, morning doses should be eliminated first.

Conversion of other opioids (e.g., codeine, hydrocodone, meperidine) to sustained-release morphine sulfate or oxycodone hydrochloride preparations can be made using tables in the *Physicians' Desk Reference.*

No detoxification from opioids can ever be free of discomfort. Moreover, many withdrawal symptoms persist for several weeks after the cessation of opioid use, no matter how prolonged the taper. Various adjunctive agents can be used for added relief of symptoms.

Clonidine reduces sympathetically mediated withdrawal symptoms such as tremulousness, sweating, and rhinorrhea. Clonidine can cause marked postural hypotension, so orthostatic vital signs should be monitored at the outset of treatment. (For this reason, too, clonidine should be given with caution to patients who are on other agents that cause adrenergic blockade.) Start clonidine with two 0.1-mg transdermal patches. If this dose produces hypotension or other unwanted effects (e.g., tiredness, nausea), one patch can be removed. If 0.2 mg proves inadequate, a third 0.1-mg patch can be added. Each patch can be worn for up to a week, and the dosage should be subsequently tapered by 0.1 mg/week to discontinuation.

Dicyclomine hydrochloride, 10 mg po q6h prn, can be given to alleviate abdominal cramping and diarrhea. Kaopectate, 30 cc po after loose bowel movements, is also a useful adjunct.

During opioid detoxification, the physician should obtain urine toxicology screens every other day, if not every day, to determine whether the patient is taking unprescribed opioids or other drugs. If so, outpatient detoxification should be viewed as unsuccessful, and detoxification in a medically supervised residential treatment setting recommended. In my view, patients should be given only one chance at outpatient opioid detoxification.

Benzodiazepines and Barbiturates. Withdrawal can occur even when the patient has taken benzodiazepines, especially short-acting ones such as alprazolam and triazolam, in therapeutic doses for only a few months. A primary concern in treating benzodiazepine and all other sedative dependence is preventing major withdrawal phenomena: delirium, hallucinosis, and seizures.

Because of the low abuse liability of benzodiazepines, most patients dependent on one have been prescribed it for anxiety, insomnia, or epilepsy. Occasionally, patients use illegally obtained benzodiazepines to reduce withdrawal from alcohol or opioids and may, in the process, become dependent on them. I recommend that patients be detoxified from benzodiazepines if they have been taking them on a daily basis as their mainstay to control psychiatric symptoms (e.g., anxiety) for longer than six months. If the drug was prescribed by a psychiatrist, the primary care physician should contact the psychiatrist to clarify the ongoing role of the medication in the patient's long-term treatment plan. I also suggest detoxification from benzodiazepines if the daily dosage exceeds that recommended by the *Physicians' Desk Reference* or if patients experience withdrawal symptoms at any dosage. While many benzodiazepine withdrawal symptoms mimic those of anxiety disorders, some are quite different. Included among this latter group are marked tremulousness, cognitive impairment, illusions, hallucinations, paresthesias of the limbs and face, fasciculations, and significant elevations in blood pressure and pulse.

The general considerations for determining whether benzodiazepine or other sedative withdrawal can be accomplished safely on an outpatient basis are the same as those for alcohol detoxification. To minimize the chance of missing dependence on several substances or mistaking hyperthyroidism for sedative withdrawal, the primary care physician should obtain a urine toxicology screen, blood alcohol level, and thyroid function tests. Any psychiatric or neurologic disorder for which the patient initially began taking benzodiazepines must be closely monitored during detoxification.

The starting dose for any sedative taper is often difficult to determine because patients may not accurately report the amount of medication they have been taking—sometimes they have lost count of the pills; at other times they are embarrassed. A starting dose is best determined by contacting the patient's pharmacy or looking at the patient's prescription bottle, ascertaining how many pills were taken during the most recent weeks of usage, and then estimating an average daily dosage.

In benzodiazepine detoxification, it is wise to use the "offending agent" whenever possible because many benzodiazepines have only partial cross-tolerance (see below). This principle should, however, be balanced against a desire to use a benzodiazepine with a long enough half-life to ensure a smooth taper. For purposes of outpatient detoxification, diazepam can be

used with patients dependent on chlordiazepoxide hydrochloride or oxazepam. Clonazepam is often used for detoxification from alprazolam or triazolam, but clonazepam has such a long half-life (48–72 hours) that tapers
can take several months. Clonazepam should be prescribed with great caution for elderly patients and for those with impaired hepatic function. The
starting total daily dose of clonazepam is the cumulative dose required to
ameliorate a pulse greater than 90, nervousness, or tremulousness, giving 1
mg of clonazepam po q2h prn after stopping the benzodiazepine to be withdrawn. If more than 4 mg of clonazepam are required within 24 hours, the
physician should conclude that detoxification with clonazepam substitution
cannot be safely done in a primary care outpatient setting. In general, I recommend psychiatric referral for patients who cannot be tapered off alprazolam or triazolam by the primary care physician.

Barbiturate detoxification usually can be best accomplished by substi-
tuting phenobarbital for shorter-acting barbiturates by virtue of its excellent
cross-tolerance. The acute pharmacologic effect of 30 mg of phenobarbital
is roughly equivalent to that of 50 mg of butabarbital sodium or 100 mg of
secobarbital sodium. The duration of action of phenobarbital is approximately 12 hours, compared to 6–8 hours for butabarbital sodium and 3–4
hours for secobarbital sodium.

It is important to remember that the elimination of benzodiazepines and
barbiturates from the body is described as an inverse logarithmic function.
Thus, the time required to reduce the initial dose by 50 percent is also the
time required to reduce the then-halved dose by 50 percent. For example,
if it takes two weeks to taper the daily dose of lorazepam from 4 mg to 2
mg, it should also take two weeks to reduce the dose from 2 mg to 1 mg,
and so on. No matter how slowly a sedative taper is conducted, the final
decrement from some amount of drug to zero may precipitate abstinence
symptoms. For purposes of outpatient detoxification, I generally recommend that the starting dose of a benzodiazepine or barbiturate taper be reduced after the first seven days. If the patient's condition dictates that detoxification be carried out with dispatch, it should be done on an inpatient
basis.

As with detoxification from alcohol, adjunctive agents such as propranolol hydrochloride and anticonvulsants should be avoided because they only increase the likelihood of delirium and other complications.

The goal of detoxification from any psychoactive substance is absolute abstinence. Detoxification without structured, long-term follow-up should not be undertaken; otherwise, the dependence syndrome will be promptly reinstated.

Identifying and Neutralizing Sustaining Factors. Patients with medical or psychiatric disorders that are helped by the drug on which they are dependent may well be reluctant to undergo detoxification unless they are convinced that those disorders will be adequately treated in the process. For example, an opioid-dependent patient with chronic low back pain may refuse detoxification unless the physician proposes another approach to pain relief (e.g., nortriptyline, biofeedback, physical therapy). Women who are alcohol-dependent should be presumed to have major depression or an anxiety disorder until proven otherwise. The same is true for most benzodiazepine-dependent patients, regardless of sex.

Conventional wisdom has been that one cannot distinguish between substance-induced and primary mood disorders until patients have been abstinent for several months. However, if the depressive or anxiety states patients experience are a significant sustaining factor in their dependence, the primary care physician does not have the luxury of waiting that long. Practically speaking, most patients will relapse into alcohol or drug use if they do not receive adequate treatment for their underlying complaints after they are detoxified. With dependent patients with comorbid psychiatric disorders, then, close collaboration between the primary care physician and the psychiatrist is essential.

Extinguishing the Habit. Once detoxification and a plan to treat comorbid conditions are under way, the primary care physician should refer patients to alcohol or drug treatment programs. All such programs contain several common elements: concrete "steps" for the patient to follow; membership in a group for peer support, lessening of social embarrassment, and a large reservoir of positive reinforcement and encouragement; involvement of now-abstinent group members to serve as role models whose steps to recovery can be imitated; regular monitoring of progress; provision of strong countermotivation to relapse; recognition of achievements through milestones, anniversaries, and so forth; and regular follow-up over a period of years. (See below for descriptions of Alcoholics Anonymous and Narcotics Anonymous.)

Preventive Maintenance

Successful completion of detoxification or a time-limited treatment program (e.g., 30 days of residential treatment) does not constitute cure—an unfortunate assumption that most patients, their families, their employers, and all-too-many physicians make. It takes approximately two years for patients to establish a foothold on recovery, during which time they may have several relapses. In the first year, they must try to cope with the activities and stresses of everyday life—not to mention a calendar of holidays, birthdays, and season-specific events—without the use of alcohol or drugs. During the second year, they usually have a better idea of what to expect and what to do, having seen most situations at least once and tested various coping strategies.

It is important for patients to see the primary care physician on a weekly basis, if only for five minutes or so, during the first several months after detoxification and then perhaps on a biweekly basis during the second six months. Patients who can come for appointments on a regular basis, and not in a state of intoxication or withdrawal, have achieved 80 percent of the goal. During these visits, the physician should check for alcohol on the breath or drugs in the urine.

Alcohol. Sleep disturbance is a common complaint among recently detoxified alcoholic patients and can last for six months. The physician should not prescribe sedatives or hypnotics when this occurs. Instead, trazodone hydrochloride, starting at 50 mg qhs and increased to 300 mg qhs if necessary, should be used. Persistent insomnia is sometimes due to a mood disorder, in which case appropriate pharmacotherapy or psychiatric referral is indicated.

Disulfiram can be a useful adjunct in the prevention of alcoholic relapse. Disulfiram irreversibly inhibits aldehyde dehydrogenase, an enzyme crucial for the metabolism of alcohol. When alcohol is ingested and the enzyme is blocked, acetaldehyde accumulates in the blood and produces a reaction that includes vasodilation with cutaneous flushing, dyspnea, hyperventilation, and, if severe, hypotension, cardiac failure, and shock.

The purpose of disulfiram therapy is to help deter, not punish, drinking. Not a week goes by in which most practicing alcoholic patients do not awaken to vow that they will never drink again. Such patients should take disulfiram in the morning, when resolve is strong, to help make drinking unthinkable later in the day, when resolve weakens. Disulfiram therapy is most effective when supervised; that is, when the patient enlists the help of a family member or friend to observe the taking of the daily morning tablet. Disulfiram costs $0.75–0.95 per tablet, depending on the quantity purchased.

The usual starting dose is 250 mg qd, but this should be increased to 500 mg qd as the patient tolerates the medication. Side effects occur in 5 percent of patients taking 500 mg of disulfiram and include headache, drowsiness, mild delirium, peripheral neuropathy, and hepatotoxicity. The risk of hepatotoxicity from disulfiram is less than that from chronic alcohol use, but liver function tests should be regularly done.

Patients must not take disulfiram until they have been abstinent from alcohol for at least 24 hours. It is contraindicated in patients with significant coronary artery disease and in those taking warfarin sodium, metronidazole, phenytoin, tricyclic antidepressants, and most benzodiazepines, with whose metabolism it interferes. The physician should instruct patients to avoid not only beverage alcohol, but also other alcohol-containing substances (e.g., mouthwash, aftershave lotion, cough syrups, vinegar). Because adventuresome patients may try to see if they can drink modest amounts of alcohol while taking disulfiram, the physician should warn all patients that the onset of the acetaldehyde reaction is often delayed until an hour or more after drinking. Patients should be told to go immediately to an emergency room if they believe they are developing the reaction, which is treated with blood pressure support, oxygen, and large doses of vitamin C.

Naltrexone hydrochloride, an opioid antagonist, has recently proven a valuable adjunct in the prevention of alcoholic relapse. Evidence suggests that alcohol stimulates endogenous opiate production in the brain—a mechanism believed to be linked to the development of a "taste," if not a craving, for alcohol. Naltrexone hydrochloride diminishes this craving and even the "drinking dreams" frequently experienced by abstinent alcoholic persons. In the presence of naltrexone hydrochloride, alcohol has less of a euphoriant effect, so patients should not stop taking it if they relapse.

The usual dose of naltrexone hydrochloride is 50 mg qd. Patients taking the medication often experience initial malaise, myalgias, headache, and a mild flulike syndrome that disappears after several days. For this reason, naltrexone hydrochloride should be started at 25 mg qd for three days, followed by an increase to 50 mg qd. If patients continue to experience cravings for alcohol or "drinking dreams," the dose can be increased to as much as 200 mg per day, provided that liver enzymes are closely monitored.

Naltrexone hydrochloride is contraindicated in patients taking opioids and in those with acute hepatitis or liver failure. It should be stopped at least a week before anticipated surgery. Common side effects include appetite and weight loss and elevation of liver enzymes, which should be monitored regularly. As with disulfiram, the risk of hepatotoxicity from naltrexone hydrochloride pales by comparison to that from alcohol. Naltrexone hydrochloride can be used in concert with disulfiram. Physicians should be aware that some insurance reimbursement plans will not pay for naltrexone hydrochloride. One hopes that this situation will change as its effectiveness is more widely recognized.

Alcoholics Anonymous (AA), a nonclinical, nonprofessional self-help organization, can be very helpful to alcoholic persons. AA has no dues, and its only requirement for membership is the desire to stop drinking. AA's method is one of individual character re-formation. Most alcohol-dependent persons become so engrossed in their drinking behavior that they increasingly migrate to the fringes of family and community. AA provides 12 steps for them to learn how to reintegrate themselves into a community, starting with the AA fellowship. AA's 12 steps can essentially be condensed into four: (1) *surrender* (i.e., accepting that one has lost control over alcohol intake), (2) *confession* of one's own role in creating problems, (3) *restitution* (i.e., making amends, when possible, to those who have been neglected or harmed), and (4) *replication* (i.e., helping others do the same by becoming an AA sponsor).

The first step in AA is surrender to a "higher power." Many potential members are put off by this concept, mistakenly believing that AA will force-feed religion to them. Patients should understand that "higher power" refers only to the self-confident equanimity and strength that is possessed by members who have been in recovery for years but is lacking in actively practicing alcoholic persons.

Although patients may attend and even participate in AA meetings, they often are reluctant to obtain a sponsor. A common misconception about AA sponsors is that they serve as persons to call when one is "dying for a drink." Instead, sponsors act as role models and mentors for the 12 steps and as first confidants within the fellowship community. When patients say they are attending AA, always ask if they have sponsors. If they do not, tell them they are missing most of the benefit from membership. Sponsors should have been abstinent for at least a year, have completed their own 12-step program under sponsorship, and be of the same sex if the patient is heterosexual or of the opposite sex if the patient is homosexual. Reassure shy or suspicious patients that membership in AA is completely confidential. AA chapters exist in every U.S. county, in most small towns, and in most other Western countries. Local AA groups vary greatly. It is best to encourage patients to contact an AA central office (listed in the telephone directory) for assistance in locating an AA group in which they might initially feel more comfortable (e.g., women's groups, "first-step" groups).

AA has no general policy about the use of disulfiram, naltrexone hydrochloride, or prescribed psychotropic medicines such as lithium or antidepressants. Nevertheless, certain individual AA groups have strong views on this matter, and patients who are taking such medications can find themselves criticized in those groups. If this is the case, the patient should be encouraged to try another group. Because women are a minority in AA and because so many women who are alcohol dependent have an affective disorder or anxiety disorder requiring medication, they first should be referred to a women's group.

Narcotics Anonymous (NA) is a fellowship analogous to AA but covering all psychoactive drug use, including heroin and cocaine. Patients who do not use illicit substances fare better with AA than NA, whose membership tends to be younger and to have histories of antisocial behavior.

Cocaine. Unless medical contraindications develop, it is recommended that cocaine addicts who have done well with antidepressant medication be maintained on antidepressants for at least two years.

Opioids. Naltrexone hydrochloride is an effective adjunct in the preventive maintenance of opioid dependence. A single 50-mg dose is sufficient to give total opiate receptor blockade for over 24 hours. If patients take naltrexone hydrochloride regularly, opioids will have no effect.

Naltrexone hydrochloride therapy should not be instituted until 14–21 days after opioid detoxification, lest it precipitate withdrawal symptoms, which could then trigger relapse. As in preventive maintenance for alcohol dependence, treatment should be started at 25 mg qd for three days, followed by an increase to 50 mg qd. If the patient develops significant withdrawal symptoms at a dose of 25 mg, the starting dose should be reduced to 5 mg (given as liquid) and increased on an every-other-day basis. Naltrexone hydrochloride therapy is most effective when monitored by someone other than the patient.

Methadone maintenance programs do not promote abstinence, but rather reduction in personal and social chaos caused by drug-seeking behavior. Their principle is that a legally obtained single daily dose of this long-acting opioid can be substituted for multiple daily doses of a patient's usually illicitly obtained, short-acting opioid of choice. Methadone programs usually require daily attendance, although programs administering longer-acting preparations requiring less-frequent attendance are now under study. Because methadone programs are concentrated in urban areas, patients from rural areas who seek methadone treatment should be encouraged to travel to a program for an intake evaluation and then to decide whether they should relocate to enroll. Alternatively, they could decide on a course of detoxification followed by abstinence.

When patients want to be detoxified from methadone, the physician should always contact their methadone maintenance program, for all programs have detoxification protocols. All decisions about starting, modifying, or discontinuing methadone maintenance are best left to these specialty clinics. An all-too-frequent occurrence is that a patient who comes to a primary care physician's office seeking methadone detoxification has been dropped from a program for noncompliance.

As noted above, NA is an organization analogous to AA in all respects, except that its purview extends to all psychoactive substances. If NA is not listed in the local telephone directory, most AA offices will be able provide information on how to contact NA groups.

Benzodiazepines and Barbiturates. Patients abstaining from benzodiazepines and barbiturates should be closely monitored for reemergence and appropriate treatment of the symptoms (e.g., anxiety, depression) for which they originally took the drugs.

Other Aspects of Preventive Maintenance. Relapse prevention is at the core of preventive maintenance. During brief office visits, the physician should always ask patients about abstinence, congratulate them on their achievements and anniversaries, and ask how they are getting on with their AA or NA sponsors. The discussion should then turn to the patient's family relationships, work, and finances. When things are not going well or when the patient seems distressed for any reason, longer or more frequent visits should be scheduled. If the patient's mood remains low, the physician should consider a major depression—and psychiatric referral.

Most patients eventually will ask how long they must continue to take disulfiram or naltrexone hydrochloride. The recommended response is "Usually for two years." Patients often rationalize a desire to discontinue these medications by claiming not to want to become dependent on another drug, to which a recommended response is: "These medicines are neither habit forming nor addicting. Why tamper with success?" In these situations, the physician should ask patients whether they have been having cravings or dreams of drinking or drug taking, which an increased dose of naltrexone hydrochloride might ameliorate.

Problems Common to All Practices. Patients with a history of alcohol, benzodiazepine, or barbiturate dependency should not be given sedatives or hypnotics, which all too often are routinely ordered or automatically offered on a prn basis during acute hospitalizations. This practice should be avoided, and trazodone hydrochloride used for insomnia. Because dependence can be quickly reestablished after abstinence, patients previously dependent on benzodiazepines, barbiturates, or other sedatives should never be prescribed these agents again, even for brief periods. Similarly, patients who have been dependent on benzodiazepines should never be prescribed barbiturates, and vice versa.

Analgesic treatment after surgery or injury can be awkward with patients who were previously dependent on alcohol or opioids. The primary care physician should try prescribing nonsteroidal antiinflammatory drugs or tramadol hydrochloride before prescribing opioids. Previously alcohol-dependent patients rapidly become tolerant to analgesic doses of opioids and quickly can become opioid dependent. If they ultimately do require opioid detoxification, they often relapse into drinking afterward unless preventive measures are taken. If relapse occurs, disulfiram and naltrexone hydrochloride therapy should be vigorously instituted.

Recovering opioid addicts pose a special challenge after surgery or trauma: they have much higher opioid analgesic requirements and are often perceived as "drug seeking" when unwittingly undermedicated. If nonnarcotic analgesics prove inadequate, a short-acting opioid can be administered orally and around the clock, rather than intramuscularly or on a prn basis. Opioids given on a contingent basis or via a needle usually reawaken drug cravings in these patients. The physician should assure patients that they will not suffer, and opioid analgesia should be maintained in amounts sufficient to keep them free of pain during the acute recovery; afterward, it should be abruptly discontinued. For example, a recovering addict who requires extraction of wisdom teeth should be prescribed standing doses of a potent shorter-acting opioid (e.g., hydromorphone hydrochloride) for three days, after which it should be stopped without a taper. The abrupt discontinuation of an opioid may provoke withdrawal phenomena, even after a short course of the medication. If this occurs, adjunctive agents such as clonidine and dicyclomine hydrochloride should be used. Recovering addicts who require opioid analgesia for longer periods will require full detox-ification, as previously described, at the end of their medical or surgical care.

Again, naltrexone hydrochloride therapy should be stopped at least a week before anticipated surgery.

Anticipating Relapse. During every phase of treatment, a mutually agreed-upon relapse management plan (i.e., what the patient should do and what the physician will do) should be in place.

Relapse Management

Relapse is an essential component of the dependency syndrome. Most patients relapse several times early in the course of treatment and recovery, but relapse can occur at any time. Patients are most likely to relapse when confronted with illness or psychosocial stressors (e.g., marital problems, job loss). Relapse does not necessarily indicate lack of motivation or compli-ance, especially with patients who have expended much effort, money, and time in attempting to recover. Relapse may mean that treatment was in-complete or otherwise ineffective or that a contingency had not properly been anticipated. Most relapses arise from the loss of vigilant preventive maintenance by the patient or the physician.

Most patients are reluctant to contact their physicians at the onset of re-lapse because they are embarrassed or anticipate being chastised for non-compliance. Relapse is extremely demoralizing and is experienced by pa-tients as yet another failure. Patients and physicians both need to remember that relapse is the rule, not the exception.

Relapse always requires immediate action lest the full dependency syn-drome reinstate itself. Watchful waiting is contraindicated. If a relapse man-agement plan had previously been agreed upon, it should be promptly in-stituted; if not, the physician and patient must quickly devise one. The time frame for this intervention is days, not weeks.

The physician must identify the provocative and sustaining factors for the relapse and take steps to help the patient neutralize them. As this is being done, abstinence should be restored by ensuring that the patient is in a supervised environment, free from drink or drugs. A structured daily routine should be restored and appropriate social roles reinstated as soon as possible. Such swift and definitive measures can prevent the need for detoxification or a residential treatment program. With proper relapse management, the patient rapidly can resume the preventive maintenance mode, now buttressed against contingencies that previously had gone unanticipated or uncountered.

Most patients and physicians mistakenly believe that relapse inevitably means they must start all over from the beginning, as if recovery were a streak of consecutive days, months, or years of abstinence, which relapse puts back to zero. Such a stance demoralizes all parties and discourages and delays reentry into treatment, which in turn guarantees full reinstatement of the dependence syndrome, the need for a full course of treatment, and sometimes an overwhelming desire to give up.

A far more realistic and constructive way of viewing recovery is to encourage patients to chart the percentage of nonabstinent days per unit of time, with an ultimate goal of 100 percent. If, for example, the unit of time is a year, a drinker who goes from daily use to periods of abstinence lasting one month, three months, and seven months during a year improves from 0 to 91 percent (11 of 12 months). If that patient has two one-week relapses the following year, improvement rises to 96 percent. In this way, as long as patients have periods of abstinence, one-day "slips" or brief relapses never return them to zero improvement.

As patients proceed in their recovery, relapses become shorter and much less frequent. Each relapse should be turned into a learning experience that yields a new strategy for coping with contingencies that had not been effectively countered. With any relapse, the physician should remind patients and encourage them that, if they stick with it, they will eventually recover. Physicians, who may also get demoralized in the face of relapse, need to remember that, too.

Allocation of Time and Resources

Treating psychoactive substance use disorders requires much time, energy, and other resources. After an evaluation, diagnostic formulation, and treatment recommendations have been completed, the primary care physician should assess the patient's motivation so that the physician's time can be wisely allocated. The motivation of patients who present for treatment can be divided into three broad, but not mutually exclusive, categories.

The first category comprises persons with whom dialogues about diagnosis and treatment quickly become debates. These individuals are easily recognized because they seem to haggle over every aspect of treatment, often down to defining words. Every encounter with them feels like a struggle. They are usually interested not in how to change for the better, but in how quickly someone else (in this case, the physician) will provide relief of the physical and social consequences of their behavior. Because they can see no further, their substance use disorders are untreatable and their prognosis is poor.

The second category is composed of persons who are easy to recognize because their goal is recovery, and they will attempt anything reasonable that is asked of them. After exploring treatment options, they usually become patients by closing on a treatment plan without much negotiating. Even if they do not accept the treatment offered, the physician never finds him- or herself haggling with them. Their prognosis is good.

The third category is not as readily recognizable. These persons will attempt some of what is reasonably asked of them but seem unwilling to make a commitment to the rest. They are more like contemplative clients than patients, choosing this aspect of treatment and rejecting that. They ask many questions and are concerned about their "right" to direct how certain situations will be handled, regardless of the effect on treatment as a whole. The physician frequently finds him- or herself spending much time trying to win them over completely to patienthood. Their prognosis is fair.

Time and resources are best spent, first, by identifying, counseling, and treating persons who agree to be patients; second, by trying to convert clients into patients; and, third, by succinctly giving untreatable persons ex-

plicit instructions as to what they must do to become treatable and invit-
ing them back when they are ready to attempt treatment. Resources given
to the preventive maintenance of well-motivated patients are resources well
allocated.

Summary

Injudicious or illicit use of alcohol and other psychoactive drugs is the most
common psychiatric problem in primary care settings. Effective treatment
rests upon recognizing it promptly, developing a healthy respect for the
powerful neuropharmacologic properties of these agents, and not blaming
patients for their afflictions. Each agent's virulence derives more from its
abuse liability and withdrawal potential than from the vulnerabilities of
those it affects. Psychoactive substance use disorders are most accurately diagnosed by history. Any suspicion of alcohol or drug use should be followed
by appropriate laboratory studies, including a urine toxicology screen. The
physician should explain exactly what *dependence syndrome* or *harmful use*
means and then provide evidence for the diagnosis based on the history, examination, and laboratory findings.

All treatment plans have three essential steps: (1) stopping the drug-
taking behavior, (2) neutralizing factors that sustain that behavior, and (3)
establishing a program to extinguish the habitual aspects of the behavior.
Medical detoxification may be needed by patients likely to experience withdrawal symptoms. Detoxification should not be undertaken without a long-
term follow-up plan in place, except in medical emergencies or when withdrawal significantly compromises the treatment of other disorders. If
patients do not receive adequate treatment for their underlying complaints,
most will relapse after detoxification. Once a plan for treatment of comorbid conditions is under way, patients should be referred to drug or alcohol
treatment programs. There is no cure—only preventive maintenance—for
psychoactive substance use disorder. It takes approximately two years for
most patients to establish a foothold on recovery, during which time they
may have several relapses. Frequent, regular office visits that include monitoring for alcohol in the breath or drugs in the urine are key to preventive

maintenance. All patients should be encouraged to give Alcoholics Anonymous or Narcotics Anonymous a fair trial. Relapse prevention is at the core of preventive maintenance. A dependence syndrome can reinstate itself after only a few days of alcohol or drug use, even after years of abstinence, so physicians must exercise great caution in prescribing psychoactive drugs for patients in recovery.

REFERENCES

Agency for Health Care Policy and Research (AHCPR), U.S. Department of Health and Human Services. *Evidence Report/Technical Assessment, Number 5: Pharmacotherapy for Alcohol Dependence.* Rockville, Md.: AHCPR Publication No. 99-E004, 1999.

American Psychiatric Association. Practice Guideline for the Treatment of Patients with Substance Use Disorders: Alcohol, Cocaine, Opioids. *American Journal of Psychiatry* 152 (1995): November Supplement.

Ashton, Heather. Benzodiazepine Withdrawal: An Unfinished Story. *British Medical Journal* 288 (1984): 1135–1140.

Edwards, Griffith, and Gross, Milton M. Alcohol Dependence: Provisional Description of a Clinical Syndrome. *British Medical Journal* 1 (1976): 1058–1061.

Ewing, John A. Detecting Alcoholism: The CAGE Questionnaire. *Journal of the American Medical Association* 252 (1984): 1905–1907.

O'Brien, Charles P., and Jaffe, Jerome H., editors. *Addictive States.* Research Publications, Association for Research in Nervous and Mental Disease, Vol. 70. New York: Raven Press, 1992.

Romanoski, Alan J. Alcohol and Drug Dependence. In *The Principles and Practice of Medicine,* 23d ed., edited by John D. Stobo, David B. Hellman, Paul W. Ladenson, Brent G. Petty, and Thomas A. Traill, pp. 927–936. Stamford, Conn.: Appleton and Lange, 1998.

PART II

Neurologic Problems

EIGHT

The Screening Neurologic Evaluation

Orest Hurko, M.D.

It has been said that neurologic diagnosis is 85 percent history, 10 percent physical examination, and 5 percent ancillary testing. Thus, evaluation of the patient with a neurologic complaint starts with analysis of the patient's history. The second step is the formulation of an anatomic differential diagnosis: which area of the nervous system could be malfunctioning to give rise to the patient's symptoms? A carefully taken history will yield only a small number of anatomic hypotheses. The neurologic examination is the third step. Its purpose is to determine which of the limited number of possibilities is the most likely. Because the number of neurologic diseases is so large, it is critical for the primary care physician to follow this three-step procedure. A successful examiner must have a notion of what the anatomic possibilities might be before beginning the actual physical examination. Only by letting the history focus the examination will the physician arrive at a clinical diagnosis that can become an efficient tool.

For the primary care physician, it is sufficient to know the features of the commonly encountered clinical situations described in this book as well as a few basic neurologic tests described in this chapter. With this information, it should be possible to decide when to refer to a specialist and when to initiate management without such consultation.

What anatomic hypotheses need to be considered? For a first approximation, it is sufficient to consider six major neuroanatomic possibilities. Working from the periphery inward, the physician should consider whether the primary problem is in (1) skeletal muscle, (2) the neuromuscular junction, (3) peripheral nerves, (4) the spinal cord, (5) the posterior fossa (brainstem and cerebellum), or (6) the telencephalon (cortex, deep white matter, or basal ganglia). One should always consider a seventh anatomic category: does the problem originate outside the nervous system? The knowledge of these patterns, rather than the niceness of the neurologic examination, distinguishes the experienced practitioner from the novice.

Dysfunction in any of the six anatomic regions gives rise to a characteristic pattern of neurologic signs. Rarely, if ever, does a single sign yield a diagnosis; it is the pattern that is distinctive. The examiner's aim is to elicit signs that will distinguish between the anatomic diagnoses suggested by the history. Working this way, the clinician will become aware of the importance of even subtle signs—if they are part of a larger pattern that fits the patient's clinical situation.

How are these patterns to be constructed? As in all physical diagnosis, the examiner begins with vital signs and direct examination of the part of the body where the symptoms originate (e.g., the stiff neck, the painful back, the weak or painful limb). The neurologist adds to this basic approach six specific examinations: (1) mental state, (2) cranial nerves, (3) motor system, (4) reflexes, (5) coordination, and (6) sensation.

Basic Anatomic Patterns

Myopathy

Myopathy yields the simplest of patterns: there is dysfunction of only the motor system. There is no abnormality of sensation, coordination, reflexes, the cranial nerves themselves, or mental state. With few exceptions, the weakness is symmetric and most marked proximally: lifting the arms over the shoulders, using the hip muscles to arise from a squat or a chair. Distal muscles are relatively spared.

There are only a few exceptions. In some myopathies, there may be false "cranial nerve signs": weakness of the extraocular muscles in thyrotoxic myopathy, weakness of neck flexion or extension in polymyositis. Although there are no sensory deficits in pure myopathies, some myopathies may be associated with an aching pain or muscle tenderness. Finally, if myopathic weakness is extremely severe, it may be impossible for the physician to detect a reflex jerk.

Neuromuscular Junction Disorders

Neuromuscular junction disorders, too, give rise to a simple pattern, limited to dysfunction of the motor system. Unlike myopathy, myasthenia gravis is a disorder of fatigue more than of constant weakness. Symptoms fluctuate and are worse at the end of the day. Signs may become apparent only after repeated testing that fatigues what may initially be an excellent response. Invariably there are cranial nerve signs—weakness of facial and extraocular muscles, including the eyelids. In early cases, these can be very asymmetric.

Peripheral Nerve Disorders

Complete disruption of a peripheral nerve abolishes sensation and leads to flaccid paralysis of only those muscles that the nerve supplies. Partial lesions give rise to a lesser degree of altered sensation and milder weakness, frequently with pain or tingling. Familiar examples are compression of the median nerve in the carpal tunnel and disc herniation onto an exiting nerve root. Unless a physician does these sorts of examinations daily or is blessed with an unusually good memory, he or she will have to examine for such patterns with an anatomic chart open at the examining table.

In contrast to such focal dysfunction, generalized peripheral neuropathies tend to impair the longest nerve fibers. Unlike the proximal weakness seen in myopathies, the weakness is mostly distal, and there is also distal sensory loss. Typically, reflexes are diminished or absent.

The primary care physician should keep in mind two considerations. First, unlike the complete sensorimotor dysfunction resulting from complete transection, symmetric neuropathies often give partial abnormalities. Small-fiber neuropathies, as seen in diabetes or alcoholism, selectively impair pain and temperature sensation, leaving relatively intact vibratory sensation, reflexes, and motor power (all subserved by large nerve fibers). Second, most of the cranial nerves are peripheral nerves that happen to be in the head. They may be involved in focal or symmetric dysfunction, just like their counterparts in the arms and legs.

Myelopathy

Complete transection of the spinal cord gives rise to an unmistakable pattern: loss of sensation and strength below the level of the lesion. Bowel and bladder control is lost. After acute transection, "spinal shock" temporarily causes flaccidity and areflexia. In contrast, chronic partial lesions cause spasticity and hyperreflexia. In partial progressive lesions, muscle tone is affected more than strength. For example, most patients with cervical stenosis will develop some degree of spasticity and hyperreflexia before weakness or sensory abnormality is evident. Asymmetric lesions give rise to a pathognomonic pattern: ipsilateral decreased large-fiber sensation on the side of the weakness below the level of the lesion, with decreased small-fiber sensation contralaterally.

Posterior Fossa Lesions

The hallmark of a brainstem lesion is cranial nerve dysfunction ipsilaterally, with contralateral long tract signs—spasticity, weakness, and sensory loss of the limbs. If there is interruption of the midline reticular activating system, there will be stupor or coma. Involvement of the cerebellum or its connecting fibers will cause ataxia. It is important to remember that cranial nerves I (the olfactory nerve) and II (the optic nerve) are not really peripheral nerves, nor do they enter the posterior fossa. Dysfunction of smell or visual fields implies dysfunction above the level of the brainstem.

Forebrain Lesions

Complete dysfunction of one cerebral hemisphere causes contralateral spastic paralysis, impaired sensation, and visual field loss. Mental state is impaired: language is lost if the dominant (almost always the left) hemisphere is involved; spatial orientation and arithmetic ability are lost with nondominant hemispheral lesions. Consciousness is not impaired in strictly unilateral lesions.

In partial lesions, the same general patterns apply, subject to a few simple qualifications. First, motor control and expressive language are functions of the frontal lobe. Bodily sensations, receptive language, and vision are expressed more posteriorly. Second, the homunculus is spread widely over the gyri of the sensorimotor cortex but quite concentrated in the deep projecting fibers. Accordingly, some cortically based lesions will preferentially involve the face, hand, and arm, others preferentially the leg. If strength or sensation is equally impaired in the face, arm, and leg of one side of the body, this implies a lesion in the deep white matter. Third, if there is impairment of the basal ganglia rather than the cortically based pyramidal system, there will be an "extrapyramidal syndrome" of rigidity, dystonia, or choreoathetosis rather than spastic weakness. Finally, the projections of the optic nerve traverse all lobes of the cortex except the frontal lobe—upper visual fields traversing the temporal lobe, lower fields the parietal lobe, with both ending in the occipital lobe.

Neurologic Examination

Mental State Examination

The purpose of a mental state examination is to determine whether there is diffuse or localized impairment of forebrain structures. The physician first judges whether the patient is alert and attentive, both by observation during the preliminaries to the examination and formally by asking for serial subtraction of 7 from 100 (provided that the patient does not have an expressive dysphasia). More refined localization is possible only if the patient is alert. If the patient is not alert, this implies dysfunction of either the brainstem or both cerebral hemispheres.

Next, the examiner instructs the patient to remember three unrelated objects, checking initially to make sure they were registered and again in five minutes to see if they were remembered. Selective impairment of memory implies dysfunction of both hippocampi or their associated fiber tracts.

Language is tested by listening for errors of expression, comprehension, repetition, naming, reading, and writing. Selective language dysfunction implies dysfunction of the dominant (usually left) cerebral hemisphere. Difficulty in producing speech but not in comprehension is an expressive aphasia, resulting from dysfunction of the dominant frontal lobe. Impaired comprehension with preservation of fluent though nonsensical speech is a receptive aphasia, resulting from dysfunction of the dominant parietal lobe. Spatial orientation, a test of nondominant hemispheral function, is demonstrated by copying of a figure or drawing of a clock, location of cities on a map drawn by the patient, and explanation of directions from home to a familiar destination, such as a shopping center or workplace.

Dysfunction of the prefrontal cortex may be manifested only by errors of judgment or planning, tested crudely at the bedside by asking what one would do in a theater fire. If a history of isolated personality change raises concern for prefrontal dysfunction, this may need to be pursued further by formal neuropsychiatric evaluation.

Further details on examination of mental state are given in Chapter 1. The Mini-Mental State Examination described in that chapter permits a rapid survey of many areas of cognition, as well as the generation of a summary score that is particularly suitable for description of patients with diffuse global impairment of cognitive function, as occurs in delirium or dementia.

Cranial Nerves

Cranial nerve (CN) I transmits the sense of smell from the nose to the base of the frontal lobe. It is rarely tested. However, unilateral loss of olfaction of a nonirritating stimulus, such as a sniff of instant coffee, would be a valuable sign of dysfunction of the prefrontal area, which is otherwise clinically silent except for neuropsychiatric disturbance.

In contrast, CN II, which mediates vision, is a workhorse in most neurologic examinations. Optic nerve function is tested by best-corrected visual acuity of each eye tested separately. Subtle lesions are detected more reliably without specialized ophthalmologic equipment by the "swinging flashlight" test—looking for paradoxical dilation of the pupil when illuminated by a flashlight rapidly swung over from the other eye. Color plates of the type used for testing color blindness are equally sensitive in detecting unilateral optic nerve dysfunction. Visual field testing is crucial. For neurologic diagnosis, it is sufficient for the physician to test all four quadrants of each eye separately, most conveniently by counting fingers, using the eye of the examiner to control for maintenance of fixation and placement of targets. Sensitivity can be increased by presenting fingers rapidly or by asking if the color of a red test object becomes less vivid in certain quadrants. Double simultaneous stimulation, with fingers presented in two different quadrants, will determine if there is visual field neglect due to a parietal lobe lesion.

CNs III, IV, and VI, which control the pupils and the extraocular muscles, are also richly informative. Pupils should be the same size bilaterally—within half a millimeter—tested in both a dimly and a brightly illuminated room. Ptosis (drooping of the eyelid) on the same side as the small pupil indicates sympathetic nerve dysfunction; on the side of the large pupil, parasympathetic (CN III) dysfunction. Finally, the physician should check for double vision in all four quadrants; any double vision (diplopia) except at the very extremes of lateral gaze is abnormal.

Additional information can be obtained by looking for nystagmus, convergence, and smooth pursuit movements, as well as accuracy and speed of saccadic eye movements. The interpretation of these tests, as well as the use of cover-uncover tests to pinpoint the site of the lesion, are specialist skills, however.

CN V controls sensation on the face as well as the muscles that open and close the jaw. Sensory function is evaluated conveniently on all three sectors of the face by inquiring about the relative coldness of a tuning fork applied to either side of the face. Clenching and opening the jaw tests motor function; asymmetric opening indicates pterygoid weakness. When the teeth are clenched, the masseter muscle can be felt tensing and bulging under the cheek. A brief palpable delay in tensing of the masseter against contralateral control is a sensitive indicator of malfunction. The jaw jerk is a simple monosynaptic reflex mediated at the level of the pons; an absent jaw jerk in the presence of hyperactive tendon jerks implies pyramidal dysfunction between the pons and the fifth segment of the cervical cord. Testing of the corneal reflex is easy to perform but a bit more complex to interpret. This is a test of the sensory portion of CN V and the motor function of CN VII. The corneal reflex is elicited by placing a cotton swab on the cornea (not the white sclera) while the patient averts his or her gaze upward. Failure of either eye to blink with corneal touch implies a sensory lesion in CN V. Failure of an eye to blink with stimulation of either cornea implies a motor lesion of CN VII.

Besides the corneal reflex, CN VII controls the muscles of facial expression as well as taste on the front of the tongue. Additional tests include assessment of strength in each of three divisions: frontalis, by counting the number of furrows on the forehead when the patient looks up; orbicularis oculi, by ipsilateral enlargement of the palpebral fissure and by inability to keep the eye shut when the examiner vigorously tries to force both eyes open; orbicularis oris, by inability to keep the lips shut against the efforts of the examiner and inability to keep the cheeks puffed up with air when the examiner presses them closed. Weakness of all three divisions indicates a lower motor lesion. Sparing of the frontalis and relative sparing of the orbicularis oculi imply an upper motor neuron lesion, above the level of the pontomedullary junction. Asymmetry of the nasolabial fold is common in healthy individuals and therefore is not useful for localization.

CN VIII mediates hearing and vestibular function. The patient should hear lightly rubbed fingers well and equally at either ear. Only if there is asymmetry is it worthwhile to proceed to Rinne and Weber tests to distinguish conductive and sensorineural loss. Unilateral lesions cause asymmetric nystagmus, most marked when the patient tries to look away from the affected side.

Unilateral diminution of the gag reflex is a reliable sign of ipsilateral dysfunction of CN IX and X, which mediate sensation in the throat, the voice box, and the viscera in the chest and abdomen.

CN XI controls the sternocleidomastoids, which should tense equally when the patient leans his or her forehead forcefully against the examiner's hand. It also controls the trapezius, which should keep the shoulders level and elevate the shoulders with equal rapidity when the patient shrugs.

CN XII controls strength and muscle bulk of the tongue, which the patient should protrude in the midline and apply with equal vigor on the inside of the cheek against the resistance of the examiner's hand placed alongside.

Motor Examination

The physician should assess the bulk, tone, and spontaneous activity of the muscles before formally testing their strength. Atrophy, a useful sign of a chronic lower motor neuron lesion, is most easily appreciated by concavity of the first dorsal interosseous on the thumb side of the back of the hand and by concavities of the hypothenar and thenar eminences on the palmar aspect. With practice, the physician can appreciate flattening of the normally rounded deltoid and unusual prominence of the tibia with atrophy of the peroneal muscles. Elsewhere, it is important to measure circumference with a tape measure, making careful use of bony landmarks and comparison with the contralateral side.

Tone is initially assessed by watching the patient's posture when walking. Scissoring of the legs implies pyramidal spasticity—dysfunction of the upper motor neuron or its projection into the spinal cord. Next, the patient bends the arm at the elbow and is told to relax, while the examiner holds the wrist and rapidly extends the arm. A spastic "clasp knife" catch indicates pyramidal dysfunction; constant "lead pipe" resistance indicates extrapyramidal rigidity; resistance increasing to match the efforts of the examiner is *gegenhalten,* usually implying diffuse cortical dysfunction. Spasticity of the legs is further examined with the patient supine and instructed to relax the legs. If tone is normal, the heel should drag the table while the examiner quickly lifts the knee upward.

Spontaneous movement is assessed with the patient at rest and maintaining fixed posture. Fasciculations are spontaneous visible jerks of individual muscles, too small to cause motion across a large joint. Fasciculations can be elicited by slapping the muscles before observation. When associated with weakness and atrophy, they are a useful sign of lower motor neuron dysfunction. As an isolated sign, they are not important, being seen in many individuals otherwise well. Tremors, as well as other abnormal movements and postures, are discussed in Chapter 14.

Only after these observations should the physician assess strength. The choice of muscles to be tested depends on the anatomic hypotheses the examiner is trying to resolve. It is best to begin with two screening exams. The patient holds his or her arms extended in front of him or her. If there is weakness because of a lesion in the central nervous system or dysfunction of any but the most distal motor nerves, the weak arm will show a pronator drift (i.e., the arm outstretched palm up will rotate inward toward a palm-down position). A similar test of the legs is made with the patient lying on his or her back and then instructed to lift the extended legs off the table quickly. The weak leg will lag behind the stronger one.

For many purposes, it is sufficient to confine formal muscle testing to flexion and extension across the major joints of each limb, comparing one side against the other. The examiner should resist such movements with an equally matched muscle of his or her own. A standoff is rated as a normal 5, victory by the examiner against palpable resistance by the patient is 4, inability to offer resistance but ability to overcome gravity is 3, a full range of motion in the absence of gravity is 2, only a flicker of motion is 1, and no motion is 0. Rarely are finer gradations very useful. Minor degrees of weakness in the legs can be missed when they are pitted against the smaller arm muscles of the examiner. To detect minor degrees of weakness in the legs, the physician must observe the patient arise from a full squat, hop on either leg, and step onto a chair.

More detailed motor examinations are required for the resolution of finer anatomic hypotheses, such as the distinction between a carpal tunnel syndrome and a cervical radiculopathy. Such examinations require specialist knowledge or reference to a table of muscle tests during the exam, with the physician remembering that the overall pattern, rather than fine gradations of power for each muscle, is paramount.

Reflexes

Testing tendon jerks is useful only if the patient is properly positioned because the strength of the response depends on the tension of the muscle before the tendon is struck. The tendon must be struck forcefully and quickly, in a reproducible manner, most conveniently using a long-handled reflex hammer rather than the more technically demanding short-handled "tomahawks." The physician should strike the biceps with the patient's elbow bent at about a right angle. Sometimes it is necessary to try minor variations of this position for optimal response, with comparison to the response of the similarly placed contralateral limb. The knee jerk is most easily elicited with the patient sitting and the lower leg dangling. Knee jerks are greatly diminished or absent when the leg is fully extended. This diminution can be exploited when comparing the relative intensity of two hyperactive jerks in a spastic patient. The ankle jerk is tested slightly dorsiflexed with gentle upward pressure on the bottom of the foot applied by the examiner while the Achilles tendon is struck. In difficult cases, it is best to have the patient kneel during this maneuver.

In all difficult cases, the physician should undertake the maneuvers with a distracting Jendrassik maneuver: asking patients to clench their teeth when the physician is testing their arms and to squeeze their hands together when the physician is testing their legs—before a tendon jerk can be pronounced absent. A simple rating scale suffices: 0 for absent, 1 for diminished, 2 for normal, 3 for increased, 4 for pathologically increased (with clonus). Clonus is sometimes spontaneously observed, but it is more often elicited by rapid passive dorsiflexion at the ankle or after tapping with a tendon hammer.

The plantar response is examined by carefully stroking the lateral sole of the foot with a key, looking for the pathological extension of the great toe with flexion of the others. The physician must take care to distinguish false positives, with all toes extending in withdrawal, and false negatives, with elicitation of a tonic grasp reflex from too medially placed a stroke.

Pathological increase of reflexes indicates an upper motor neuron lesion; diminution or absence implies a lower motor neuron lesion. The only exceptions are the transient loss or diminution of reflexes from catastrophic acute interruption of the pyramidal tracts, as happens in acute cord transections ("spinal shock") or massive ischemic strokes.

Coordination

Coordination tests are tests of the cerebellum and its connections. The midline cerebellum mediates coordination of the trunk; the lateral cerebellum, that of the ipsilateral arm and leg. Each must be tested separately.

Walking a straight line, heel to toe, is a stringent test of midline coordination, as is standing one foot in front of the other. Less difficult is standing with the feet next to each other. Individuals with severe midline deficits cannot pass the easiest of these tests—sitting on the examining table without weaving.

Each of these midline tests can be performed with the eyes closed, as in the classic Romberg test. Successful performance with eyes open means that the cerebellar circuits are functioning. To do so, they must integrate information from at least two of the three cardinal orienting modalities: vision, sensory information about the position of the body, and vestibular function. Subsequent failure with eyes closed means that at least one of the other two modalities is compromised. In most such cases, proprioception is diminished because of dysfunction in the posterior columns of the spinal cord.

Ataxia is tested in the arms by the finger-to-nose test and in the legs by the heel-to-shin test. Subtle ataxia of the upper limb can be detected by having the patient tap his or her index finger rapidly on the crease of the thumb.

Coordination testing is part of the cranial nerve examination as well. Slurring of speech or jerky or inaccurate eye movements can indicate impairment of cerebellar function.

Sensation

Testing of sensation is the last part of the examination and is the most difficult for both the examiner and the patient. Fatigue by both parties prevents anything other than selective testing. More than any other part of the examination, testing of sensation must be focused to resolve any anatomic hypotheses remaining after the history and previous examination. For example, sensory loss extending from the palm to the forearm would support a C8 radiculopathy rather than a carpal tunnel lesion; a distinct spinal level to pinprick would distinguish a spinal lesion from a lesion between both cerebral hemispheres.

In most circumstances, it suffices to test vibratory sensation (a large-fiber modality) and temperature sensation (a small-fiber modality). The physician compares an affected area with a control area—right to left, in the case of asymmetric complaints, or proximal to distal. Reference to a diagram placed next to the patient on the examining table is indispensable to all but the most accomplished specialists when trying to sort out radicular or peripheral nerve lesions.

REFERENCES

Alpers, Bernard J., and Mancall, Elliot L. *Essentials of the Neurological Examination.* Philadelphia: F. A. Davis, 1971.

Heilman, Kenneth M.; Watson, Robert T.; and Greer, Melvin. *Handbook for Differential Diagnosis of Neurologic Signs and Symptoms.* New York: Appleton-Century-Crofts, 1977.

NINE

Weakness

Richard O'Brien, M.D.

Many patients will complain to their primary care physician that they are weak. The complaint is not only common but also nonspecific. Some patients will have true muscular weakness: an inability to generate sufficiently forceful muscle contractions for walking, carrying, or lifting. Other patients will be complaining of malaise or fatigue rather than true muscular weakness.

Evaluation of the patient with either localized or generalized weakness is fairly simple, once the physician is convinced of the existence of an organic neurologic process. When evaluating a patient complaining of weakness, however, the physician must consider several common nonneurologic processes before embarking on a neuromuscular evaluation. These conditions include pain, disuse, and embellishment.

Neurologic Disorders Associated with Weakness

Weakness can be either asymmetrically localized to one part of the body or generalized. Weakness limited to a few muscle groups of one limb can result from a lesion of a nerve root exiting the spine, the lumbar or brachial plexus at the base of the limb, or a single peripheral nerve within the affected limb itself. Nerve root disease is often associated with pain in the back or neck and is discussed in Chapter 11. Compression of single peripheral nerves is frequently associated with numbness or tingling and is discussed in Chapter 13. Weakness affecting one side of the body results from lesions of the spinal cord or brain. When this occurs abruptly, it is most often due to a stroke.

More difficult to recognize is generalized weakness resulting from neuromuscular disease or cervical stenosis. Neuromuscular diseases are rare. Unlike acute strokes or painful compressive neuropathies, they tend to be symmetric, insidious in onset, and thus easily disregarded in the early stages.

Myopathies

Myopathies are diseases of muscle. They include *inflammatory* myopathies, such as polymyositis, dermatomyositis, and inclusion body myositis. The hallmark of these diseases is an immune attack on muscle similar to that of rheumatoid arthritis and lupus on joints. Inflammatory myopathies respond to treatment with immunosuppressive drugs, such as prednisone and methotrexate. The *toxic* myopathies have a clinical presentation similar to that of inflammatory myopathies but result from the use of drugs such as alcohol, colchicine, prednisone, azidothymidine (AZT), and HMG-CoA reductase inhibitors. *Inherited* myopathies usually start at a younger age than do either inflammatory or toxic myopathies. The most common genetic myopathies are Duchenne and Becker muscular dystrophy, which are X-linked; myotonic dystrophy, which is autosomal dominant; and fascioscapulohumeral dystrophy, which also is autosomal dominant.

Neuropathies

Neuropathies are diseases that affect peripheral neurons by damaging either the nerve itself (axonal neuropathies) or its myelin sheath (demyelinating neuropathies). Distinction of axonal and demyelinating neuropathies often requires nerve conduction tests. *Axonal* neuropathies are most commonly caused by metabolic derangements such as diabetes, renal failure, or liver disease. *Demyelinating* neuropathies are usually immune mediated. These include an acute monophasic illness (Guillain-Barré syndrome) and a chronic relapsing form (chronic inflammatory demyelinating polyneuropathy). Both axonal and demyelinating neuropathies can also be the result of autosomal dominant diseases.

The patient with a peripheral neuropathy has distal weakness and atrophy (ankle flexors and extensors), distal (stocking-glove) sensory loss, diminished reflexes (especially at the ankles), and normal cranial nerve (bulbar) function. Once the physician suspects a neuropathy, nerve conduction testing is indicated to separate axonal from demyelinating neuropathies. Therapeutic options are limited to the treatment of any underlying metabolic diseases in axonal neuropathies and immune suppression in nongenetic demyelinating neuropathies.

Neuromuscular Junction Diseases

Disordered function of the neuromuscular junction (NMJ) usually results from myasthenia gravis, an autoimmune disease characterized by antibodies to the nicotinic acetylcholine receptor, which mediates transmission between nerve and muscle. This disease can be associated with malignant thymoma, so a chest computed tomogram (CT) is crucial in these patients. Both myasthenic patients and those with myopathies can present with proximal muscle weakness. Patients with myasthenia almost invariably have cranial nerve (bulbar) signs such as ptosis, diplopia, and facial weakness. Elevation of blood levels of creatine kinase is not a feature of myasthenia gravis but can be associated with certain myopathies. Another neuromuscular junction disease is Lambert Eaton syndrome, which is clinically similar to myasthenia gravis but is associated with antibodies to the presynaptic calcium channels and malignant small-cell cancer of the lung.

Motor Neuron Diseases

Motor neuron diseases are almost exclusively due to amyotrophic lateral sclerosis (ALS), a sporadic and rare condition that is easily diagnosed because it is a disease of spinal and cortical motor neurons. This combination causes the classic picture of lower motor neuron signs (atrophy, fasciculations), as well as upper motor neuron signs (brisk reflexes and upgoing toes). Sensation is normal, as this is strictly a disease of the motor system. Its cause is unknown.

Although ALS is rare, it is rather easy to diagnose because of its unique combination of signs. The weakness is associated with lower motor neuron signs (atrophy, fasciculations) due to the death of lower motor neurons and brisk rather than depressed reflexes due to the death of upper motor neurons. Recent clinical trials have shown that the clinical course of ALS can be slowed with riluzole.

Cervical Spine Disease

Cervical spine disease in elderly patients is most commonly caused by progressive arthritic narrowing of the spinal column. This is worsened by falls that cause hyperextension injuries, further compressing the cervical cord. Cervical myelopathies cause exclusively upper motor neuron weakness (brisk reflexes, upgoing toes) but also cause bladder difficulties (by interrupting descending tracts) and sensory loss (by affecting the posterior columns). Cervical spine disease can also result from tumor or injury. In younger patients, spinal cord disease can be caused by multiple sclerosis or isolated transverse myelitis, an acute immune-mediated process associated with cells in the cerebrospinal fluid. Transverse myelitis differs from spondylytic cervical myelopathy in its acute onset, younger age, and cellular cerebrospinal fluid. Usually, it occurs in the thoracic, rather than the cervical, spine.

Like myopathies, cervical spine disease presents with proximal weakness. However, upper motor neuron signs are usually present (spasticity, brisk reflexes, upgoing toes), and sensory changes can be prominent (vibratory sensory loss, proprioceptive loss). Indeed, the spasticity and sensory changes may be more troublesome than the weakness. Treatment of cervical myelopathies involves surgical decompression.

Initial Evaluation

History

As with all of medicine, evaluation of weakness begins with a careful history. The first point to be clarified is what the patient means when he or she complains of weakness. Does she mean that she is "too washed out" to carry on with daily activities? Alternatively, is the strength of her muscles failing? The best way to make this distinction is to determine what specific activities cause problems. The answers to this question will also provide insight as to which muscle groups may be at fault. Weakness of proximal muscles around the shoulders makes it difficult to reach up; it will be difficult to lift a container onto a shelf or to comb one's hair. Proximal weakness of the leg muscles makes it difficult to ascend stairs or to arise from a chair or a toilet seat. Distal weakness of the hands may be first noticed as difficulty opening jars, manipulating keys, using cutlery, or buttoning buttons. Distal weakness of the foot usually manifests itself as tripping or unexpected falls on rough terrain because of a foot drop.

Associated symptoms are critically important. Significant pain or antecedent injury is frequently useful to the establishment of a diagnosis, as discussed in Chapters 10 and 11. In addition, one must remember that patients cannot exert full muscular power if attempting to do so causes pain. Involuntary reflexes prevent the exertion of full effort across a painful joint and may lead to a misperception of neuromuscular disease. The time course of the patient's symptoms is also critical to diagnosis.

Acute Weakness (1–2 weeks). In the evaluation of acute generalized weakness, the diagnosis of exclusion is always Guillain-Barré syndrome (GBS). GBS is an acute demyelinating neuropathy associated with diminished reflexes, sensory changes, and weakness. This is an important diagnosis, as the patient's condition can rapidly deteriorate, resulting in respiratory failure within 48 hours. Rapid diagnosis is mandatory because GBS responds well to treatment with plasmapheresis or intravenous immunoglobulin if instituted in a timely fashion. Therefore, the primary care physician should immediately refer any acutely weak patient with absent reflexes and sensory complaints for urgent expert evaluation and treatment.

The differential diagnosis of acute weakness includes spinal cord disease, either transverse myelitis or cervical cord compression. In the latter two conditions, upper motor neuron signs are usually present and the sensory exam usually shows a thoracic level rather than a stocking-glove pattern. The spinal tap in transverse myelitis often shows 20–100 white blood cells (WBCs), while in GBS there are usually no cells and an elevated protein level. Acute weakness of limbs and bulbar muscles, with dilated, nonreactive pupils, is the presentation of botulism, another rare condition requiring emergency treatment.

Chronic Weakness (weeks to months). The differential diagnosis of the patient with chronic weakness is quite broad in comparison to that of acute weakness. Diagnosis relies on a combination of the physical exam, the presence or absence of a family history of similar diseases, and the presence or absence of nerve or muscle toxins. Using the paradigm established below, a careful exam can easily categorize the chronically weak patient.

Physical Examination

Several points of the physical exam are crucial for the primary care physician approaching the patient with generalized weakness. First, the physician must determine whether the patient is exerting full power during testing of muscle strength or whether the apparent weakness simply reflects a submaximal effort. In other words, the examiner must determine whether there is true organic weakness or poor engagement of an intact neuromuscular apparatus because of either pain or other considerations, such as embellishment. Second, the physician must determine whether the pattern of proximal versus distal weakness, as given in the history, can be confirmed by direct observation. Third, the physician must determine whether there are associated abnormalities in examination of the cranial nerves (bulbar signs), reflexes, or sensation.

Neurologic and Nonneurologic Weakness. The first task of the primary care physician is to determine whether the patient's generalized weakness is likely to result from one of the neuromuscular or spinal disorders described above. Alternatively, weakness may occur in patients without neurologic disease. Such patients may be failing to exert full effort on the physical examination either to protect a painful limb or to embellish their presenting complaint.

Fortunately, the feel or pattern of weakness in neuromuscular diseases is completely different from that seen in painful conditions or that seen with embellishment. For example, a patient with a painful shoulder may complain not only of pain but also of weakness. Such a painful shoulder may result from an orthopedic condition such as arthritis or a tear of the rotator cuff. In these cases, there is no abnormality of the nervous system, but exertion of full muscular effort may be painful. Alternatively, the painful shoulder may arise from a neurologic problem such as a brachial plexopathy or cervical radiculopathy. In such cases, there will also be true organic weakness of the muscles supplied by the damaged nerves. The distinction between these often depends on whether there is organic weakness, common in neurologic processes but not in the purely orthopedic disorders.

In neuromuscular disorders, the weakness is quite characteristic. The examiner will feel a smooth, uniform reduction in strength. In painful conditions, the pattern is that of "give-way" weakness, which feels quite ratchety. A similar pattern of ratchety, "give-way" weakness is seen in embellishment. This happens because nonneurologic weakness results from alternating periods of 100 percent strength and 0 percent strength. If I asked you to act weak, this is how you would do it, and it would be immediately obvious. (Try it!) The smooth, uniform reduction of strength seen in organic weakness cannot be mimicked.

The second clue to the neurologic etiology of weakness is associated changes in the neurologic examination, particularly the reflexes. In most cases, neurologic weakness is associated with changes in the reflexes of the affected limb compared to the nonaffected limb. In stroke or spinal cord disease (upper motor neuron disease), reflexes are increased. In contrast, in radiculopathy or neuropathy, reflexes are reduced compared to the uninvolved limb. Sensation, although often tested, can be a difficult tool for the distinction of neurologic and nonneurologic processes, since it is too subjective. Sometimes, in spite of the physician's best efforts, the presence or absence of neurologic weakness is still unclear. In this case, an electromyographic (EMG) test, in which a fine electrode is inserted into the muscle in question, is quite useful, as is referral to a neurologist.

Proximal versus Distal Weakness. One of the most important considerations is the distinction of proximal versus distal patterns of weakness. Proximal weakness is the hallmark of diseases of muscle (inflammatory or toxic myopathies), diseases of the neuromuscular junction (myasthenia gravis), and diseases of the cervical spine. Distal weakness is the pattern seen most often with neuropathic processes (neuropathies or ALS), since the distal portions of axons are the most vulnerable to metabolic insults. Why proximal weakness is so prominent in muscle diseases is unclear. One important confounder is that cervical myelopathies also present with proximal weakness. In this case, the associated upper motor neuron signs should allow the physician to distinguish cervical myelopathy from muscle diseases.

Formal testing of proximal strength in the arms can be done manually, evaluating the strength of the deltoids by pressing down on the patient's outstretched arms. However, manual testing of the proximal muscles in the legs may fail to detect mild degrees of weakness. Therefore, the physician must observe the patient arising from a full squat and standing up from a chair without a push with the arms. Distal strength in the hands is conveniently assessed by evaluating grip, keeping the fingers spread and extended, and by curling the tips of the fingers or thumb against the opposing strength of the examiner. Distal strength in the feet can be assessed manually or by having the patient walk on heels and on toes.

Lower versus Upper Motor Neuron Weakness. The second important distinction to be made is between lower and upper motor neuron weakness. In lower motor neuron weakness (diseases of the spinal motor neurons, such as ALS and neuropathies), there are obvious atrophy and prominent fasciculations (the aberrant discharge of motor neurons). In upper motor neuron diseases, such as cervical spine compression, there are brisk reflexes and upgoing toes. Muscle tone is increased in the arms and legs. In chronic cervical spine disease, spasticity may be more prominent than weakness. As a rule, reflexes are absent or decreased in neuropathies, normal in myopathies and NMJ problems, but increased in diseases with upper motor neuron components, such as ALS or cervical spine disease.

Bulbar Signs. The final pattern of weakness to be noted is the presence or absence of bulbar signs. These include diplopia, dysarthria, dysphagia, and ptosis. Dysphagia and dysarthria are fairly nonspecific. They can be seen in myopathies, myasthenia, and ALS. When diplopia and ptosis are present, the appropriate diagnosis is myasthenia gravis until proven otherwise.

Sensation. Much of the evaluation of sensation can often be done during history taking. It is rare to have sensory signs without sensory symptoms. The sensory exam should never be a blind expedition. Instead, it should be designed to answer a few focused questions. For instance, in the presence of a generalized weakness, the absence of significant sensory loss makes the diagnosis of neuropathy or spinal cord disease unlikely and makes a myopathy, NMJ disease, or ALS more likely. A stocking-glove pattern of sensory loss is more consistent with a neuropathy, whereas a thoracic sensory level or Brown-Séquard pattern is more consistent with a spinal cord lesion. The physician should look for patterns (i.e., the big picture) during the sensory exam and not worry about mapping out each square inch of skin (see Figure 10.1). The physician should always do the sensory exam last, when the issues are focused, or much time will be wasted. Vibratory sensation can also be useful to evaluate proprioceptive function, as it applies to neuropathies (diminished reflexes) or myelopathies (brisk reflexes).

Electrodiagnostic Tests

If neuromuscular disease is suspected on the basis of history and physical examination, electrodiagnostic testing may be useful for confirmation and refinement of the diagnosis. Nerve conduction testing and EMG should in many cases be deferred until after the neurologist has seen the patient, as he or she may want to emphasize specific aspects of the test. On the other hand, if the purpose of the EMG test is to establish whether apparent weakness is organic or due to pain or embellishment, then testing before referral may be in order.

Nerve Conduction Tests

Two important bits of information can be obtained from nerve conduction testing. When a nerve is stimulated proximally, a distal electrode records the conducted response from that nerve (motor or sensory) after a certain latency. That latency divided by the distance between the stimulating and recording electrodes gives a conduction velocity (usually 40 to 50 m/sec). This is a good indicator of the state of the myelin sheath around that nerve. The amplitude of the response (usually greater than 10 μV in a sensory nerve and greater than 4 mV in a motor nerve) is an indicator of the number of axons in that nerve. Therefore, this test is the single best way to distinguish axonal neuropathies, which are usually due to metabolic (diabetes, renal failure) or toxic (alcohol, drugs) causes, from demyelinating neuropathies, which are usually genetic or dysimmune (GBS, chronic inflammatory demyelinating polyneuropathy [CIDP]).

Electromyography

The electromyographic portion of the test looks at the pattern of motor units. A motor unit consists of a motor neuron and all the muscle cells it innervates (usually 100–400). In a typical muscle like the biceps, there are several hundred motor neurons, each of which innervates about 200 myofibers. Strength is generated by increasing the number of motor units activated for a given task. By asking the patient to activate the muscle in question, the physician can observe multiple motor units. In myopathies, the motor units shrink in size because of atrophy of muscle cells. In neuropathies, the remaining motor units become quite large because surviving neurons sprout to reinnervate muscle cells left uninnervated by dying axons. Therefore, the motor units served by the surviving axons will be larger than normal. The electromyogram is a very sensitive test for the presence or absence of neuromuscular problems and can complement the physical assessment. The only caveat is that these tests are sensitive only to diseases of muscle, peripheral nerve, or anterior horn cell; they do not detect abnormalities caused by central lesions. In upper motor neuron processes such as strokes and spinal cord disease, the motor units remain normal.

Repetitive Nerve Stimulation

A third portion of peripheral electrodiagnosis is the repetitive stimulation test. During this test, the nerve is repeatedly stimulated at 3 times per second. In diseases of the neuromuscular junction, repeated stimulation depletes the nerve terminals of acetylcholine, resulting in a decremented response that is specific for myasthenia gravis.

In actual practice, a weak patient first undergoes nerve conduction testing. If this is normal, EMG is performed to look for the presence of a myopathy (small motor units). If this is normal, repetitive stimulation is performed to evaluate the presence of myasthenia gravis. One important rule of electrodiagnostic testing is to limit the study to weak muscles because normal muscles will give normal results.

Referral to a Neurologist

As a rule, most organic weakness of neurologic origin is due to a stroke, a neuromuscular disease, or spinal cord disease. Strokes are usually fairly easy to distinguish, since they have a sudden onset and fit easily identified patterns. Recent advances in stroke management dictate prompt referral for emergency diagnosis and treatment. The primary care physician should usually refer patients with spinal or neuromuscular causes of weakness to a neurologist because their rarity makes pattern recognition somewhat more difficult. Additionally, many of these neuromuscular diseases should be treated with significant immunosuppression, itself a specialist skill.

Therefore, the role of the primary care physician is to establish the presence of organic weakness and its time course. Generalized weakness progressing over one to three weeks should be referred to an emergency room because of the possibility of spinal cord disease or Guillain-Barré syndrome. Subacute weakness should be referred, in a timely fashion, on an outpatient basis.

Summary

The initial task of the physician considering a complaint of weakness is to determine whether the patient is indeed weak or is offering a more general symptom. Characteristic patterns of weakness permit identification of the central or peripheral anatomic locus of the underlying lesion. These patterns are suggested by detailed history but should be confirmed by physical examination. Special care must be taken to appreciate the symptoms of myasthenia gravis, a disorder of fatigue in which the level of weakness can fluctuate dramatically. Most cases of true organic weakness benefit from referral for specialist care.

REFERENCE

Brooke, Michael H. *A Clinician's View of Neuromuscular Diseases.* Baltimore: Williams and Wilkins Co., 1977.

TEN

Numbness or Tingling

Vinay Chaudhry, M.D.

Numbness and tingling, particularly when painful, can be problems in their own right, from which the patient seeks relief. More often, they can raise concern about underlying disease. However, fleeting bodily sensations, some of them unpleasant, are a common part of everyday life. The likelihood of their being reported depends in part on the patient's level of self-awareness. When offered such a complaint, the primary care physician has to gauge its likely origins and then decide whether to reassure the patient, pursue further workup, refer to a specialist, or initiate treatment. It is a difficult area but one that can be made tractable with the recognition of a few cardinal patterns, chiefly anatomic.

The Phenomena of Numbness and Tingling

Normally, sensation results from stimulation—either normal or pathological—of a part of the body, which is then transmitted by a peripheral nerve to the central nervous system, which perceives and interprets the sensory message. However, injury to the nervous system can alter sensation, even without direct involvement of the body part in which the sensation is perceived. All forms of paresthesia, such as tingling, are considered positive phenomena (Table 10.1). They can result from abnormal generation of impulses in damaged nerves or abnormal processing of peripheral nerve signals by the brain or spinal cord.

On the other hand, numbness is a negative phenomenon. Patients may describe "heaviness," "deadness," or a "novocaine-like" feeling, similar to that experienced after dental work. Numbness implies that nerve fibers are

Table 10.1. Positive Sensory Phenomena

Phenomenon	Definition
Paresthesia	Any unpleasant, unusual, or abnormal sensation. Patients may describe burning, prickling, cutting pain, electric shock, tingling, pins and needles, crawling sensation, limb going to sleep, cramplike sensation, "poor circulation," or coolness.
Dysesthesia	Particularly intense and distressing or painful paresthesia
Hyperesthesia	Increased sensitivity to externally applied stimuli, usually with an unpleasant quality
Hyperpathia	Exaggerated response to a stimulus that is usually less painful. Often it is a delayed aftersensation to a repetitive stimulus.
Allodynia	Pain induced by a stimulus that is ordinarily not painful, such as light stroking of the skin or contact with clothing
Hyperalgesia	Increased sensitivity to painful stimuli
Neuralgia	Sharp, sudden, and short-lived pain
Causalgia	Sustained burning, abnormal microcirculation, and sweating after traumatic nerve injury

not conducting impulses efficiently because of either loss of nerve fibers or block of conduction. However, patients occasionally use the term *numbness* to refer to a weak or paralyzed limb with normal sensibility.

Positive and negative phenomena often coexist. Indeed, patients often find it strange that a part of the limb that is numb to touch can simultaneously register pain or other unusual sensations. In general, positive phenomena are more distressing to the patient than is numbness.

Unless a nerve is interrupted completely, the first manifestations of peripheral nerve disease are paresthesias. As the disease progresses, patients will experience both paresthesias and numbness. With some longstanding, slowly progressive neuropathies, patients may develop numbness of which they themselves are unaware until examined, without ever having experienced paresthesias.

Numbness can affect the patient in several ways. There may be gait difficulty because of inability to feel an uneven surface. There may be problems with dexterity because of inability to feel objects in the hand. In severe cases, there may be inadvertent cuts, burns, or pressure injury because of inability to perceive sharp or hot objects, ill-fitting shoes, or improperly aligned joints.

Common Patterns of Numbness and Tingling

When presented with a sensory complaint, the primary care physician must first decide whether the complaint originates from (1) the peripheral nervous system, (2) the central nervous system, (3) functional problems, or (4) a nonneurologic cause. Each of these causes gives rise to characteristic anatomic and temporal patterns that the physician should actively seek when taking the history and performing the physical examination.

Peripheral Nervous System Causes

Dysfunction of the peripheral nervous system can be due to either a *generalized* peripheral neuropathy or a mononeuropathy. An intermediate form is that of *mononeuropathy multiplex,* in which a series of individual, usually ischemic, nerve lesions may sum into a more diffuse pattern that can at times be difficult to distinguish from generalized peripheral neuropathy (Table 10.2).

Symmetric Peripheral Neuropathies. Generalized peripheral neuropathies generate the familiar symmetric stocking-glove pattern (Fig. 10.1a). Most of these disorders are length dependent—the longest nerve fibers are the most vulnerable and the first to be affected. Symptoms generally start in the toes, progress to involve the feet, ascend the legs, and then involve the fingers, progressing up to the hands and arms. These neuropathies can involve only *small fibers,* which mediate pain and temperature sensation; *large fibers,* which mediate vibratory sensation, reflexes, and motor outflow; or both. A similar pattern of numbness and tingling in hands and feet—as well as periorally—may occur with hyperventilation, although the symptoms would be transient and intermittent, occurring in all four limbs at the onset.

Mononeuropathies. Solitary lesions give rise to focal numbness, affecting only part of a limb. Complete lesions affect both large and small fibers, compromising all sensory modalities, motor power, and reflexes in the distribution of the affected nerve(s). Such lesions may involve only a single peripheral nerve (mononeuropathy), resulting from compression, ischemia,

Table 10.2. Common Causes of Numbness: Peripheral Nervous System

Pattern	Localization	Cause
Focal	Mononeuropathy	Compression, ischemia, trauma, trigeminal neuralgia
	Radiculopathy	Disc disease, osteophytes, tumors, (post)herpetic neuralgia (sensory)
	Plexopathy	Trauma, neoplasm, immune-mediated
Multifocal	Mononeuropathy multiplex	Diabetes mellitus, vasculitis, leukemia, lymphoma, leprosy
	Multilevel radiculopathy	Carcinoma
	Sensory neuronopathy	Paraneoplastic processes, Sjögren syndrome
Symmetric distal	Small-fiber neuropathy	Diabetes, alcohol-nutritional causes, amyloid, AIDS (and antiviral drugs)
	Large-fiber neuropathy	*Sensory ganglionitis:* carcinomatous, Sjögren synd.
		Demyelinating: Guillain-Barré syndrome
		Infectious: tabes dorsalis
		Toxic: pyridoxine, antineoplastic drugs

or trauma. The most common compressive (entrapment) neuropathies are listed in Table 10.3.

Mononeuropathies can also occur on the face. Repeated bouts of recurrent lancinating pain involving a single dermatome on the face are the hallmark of trigeminal neuralgia, which can be either an isolated disorder or a manifestation of multiple sclerosis or a compressive lesion.

Radiculopathies. Exquisitely painful sensory radiculopathy in the presence of vesicular lesions anywhere on the body is the hallmark of herpes zoster. Typically this occurs in one or more thoracic dermatomes of elderly individuals, but it may occur in younger individuals, particularly if they are immunosuppressed. The profoundly painful paresthesias and hyperesthesia usually subside after the vesicles clear. However, depending on the severity of the insult to the affected dorsal root ganglia, various degrees of numbness, pain, and hyperpathia can persist for months after the vesicles clear. The pain of postherpetic neuralgia is very difficult to treat. Often the most disabling feature of this syndrome is hyperpathia, in which affected patients are unable to tolerate even innocuous pressure from clothing or bed sheets.

Another cause of radiculopathy associated with pain and numbness is compression of exiting nerve roots by bulging discs or osteophytes. These can involve lumbosacral roots, as discussed in Chapter 11, or cervical roots. Among these is the important pattern of saddle anesthesia resulting from

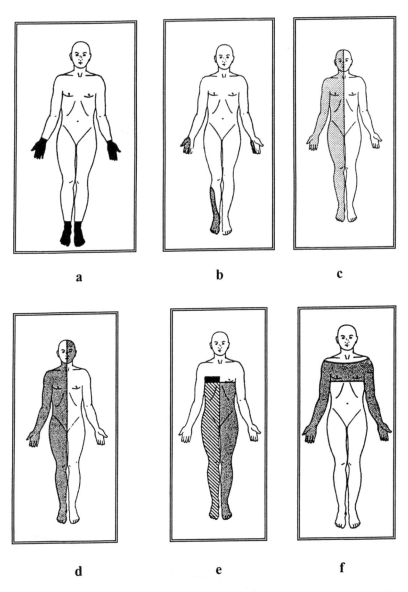

Figure 10.1. Patterns of sensory disturbance: (a) stocking-glove pattern involving distal extremities, typical of symmetric, length-dependent neuropathies; (b) mononeuropathy multiplex, one of many possible patterns resulting from involvement of multiple individual peripheral nerves; (c) ipsilateral face and body, a pattern typical of a deep hemispheral lesion involving the opposite thalamus or white matter tracts in the internal capsule; (d) face and contralateral body, a characteristic crossed pattern

Table 10.3. Entrapment Neuropathies

Symptom	Site	Paresthesia	Precipitant	Examination
Focal numbness in fingers or hand	Carpal tunnel	Thumb side of hand and fingers, sometimes extending to forearm	Sleep or repetitive hand activity	Hypesthesia on palmar surface of thumb, second finger, and third finger Weakness of thenar muscles Tinel's and Phalen's signs at wrist
	Ulnar nerve at elbow	Pinky side of hand and forearm	Flexion during sleep	Hypesthesia of pinky side of hand and fingers Weakness of interossei
	Ulnar nerve at wrist	Pinky side of hand and fingers	Repetitive hand activities, bicycling	Hypesthesia of fingers only Weakness of selected intrinsic muscles
	Thoracic outlet	Pinky side of arm, forearm, hand, and fingers	Lifting of heavy objects	Sensory loss resembling ulnar nerve, motor loss resembling median
Focal numbness in thigh or foot	Meralgia paresthetica	Anterolateral thigh	Standing or walking; recent weight gain	Hypesthesia limited to "pants pocket" distribution
	Peroneal nerve at fibular head	Top of foot	Usually acute compression; weight loss	Hypesthesia of anterolateral leg and dorsum of foot; weakness of dorsiflexion and eversion at the ankle
	Tarsal tunnel	Sole of foot, sparing heel	Prolonged standing at end of day; nocturnal	Hypesthesia on sole of foot; Tinel's sign at tarsal tunnel

resulting from a brainstem lesion involving the connections of cranial nerve V and the adjacent ascending tracts from the opposite side of the body; (e) Brown-Séquard syndrome, a pathognomic pattern resulting from hemisection of the thoracic spinal cord, interrupting the uncrossed large-fiber tracts in the posterior columns and the crossed small-fiber spinothalamic fibers; (f) suspended sensory "cape" resulting from a central cord lesion that interrupts crossing small fibers but spares posterior columns and spinothalamic tracts that had already crossed at more caudal levels. The author thanks Dr. Neil Holland for permission to modify his drawings for this figure.

compression of multiple nerve roots in the cauda equina that innervate the central part of the buttocks.

Plexopathies. A lesion of the brachial or lumbar plexus (plexopathy) will affect portions of several nerves in the arm or leg and may result in more diffuse or patchy numbness. These lesions are usually due to trauma, immune disease, or neoplasm. A detailed knowledge of the anatomy of individual nerves is important for the localization of solitary nerve lesions.

Mononeuropathy Multiplex. Mononeuropathy multiplex is easily recognized if only a few nerves are affected (Fig. 10.1*b*). Over the long term, however, it may develop into a diffuse picture that can be distinguished from distal symmetric neuropathy only by the history of abrupt, stepwise accumulation of discreet lesions of individual nerves. These usually result from small infarctions of nerves in diabetes mellitus or vasculitis, leukemia, lymphoma, or, in the developing world, leprosy. Dorsal root ganglion lesions (ganglionopathy or sensory neuronopathy) may also manifest as multifocal numbness. Paraneoplastic processes and Sjögren syndrome are among the causes of sensory neuronopathy.

Central Nervous System Causes

Altered sensation can result from lesions in the central nervous system (Table 10.4). Lesions in the *cerebral hemispheres* alter sensation on the opposite side of the body.

Lesions of the Cerebral Cortex. If the lesions are superficial, involving the cortex, the face, arm, and leg will not be affected equally because the ho-

Table 10.4. Common Causes of Numbness: Central Nervous System

Localization	Duration	Cause
Cortical	Transient	Migraine, seizure, transient ischemic attack
	Sustained	Large-vessel stroke, metastatic tumor, meningioma
Subcortical (thalamic or posterior capsule)	Sustained	Lacunar stroke, multiple sclerosis, astrocytic tumor
Brainstem	Sustained	Stroke, multiple sclerosis, tumor
Spinal cord	Sustained	Multiple sclerosis, trauma, metastatic tumor, syringomyelia

munculus representing the body extends widely over the brain surface. Transient numbness beginning in the hand or face and spreading over adjacent parts of the body in a matter of minutes is a classic prodrome of migraine. Similar spread occurring in a matter of seconds is typical of a seizure. Instantaneous numbness of face and arm lasting for minutes to hours is typical of transient ischemic attack (TIA) involving a large vessel, from either a cardiac embolus or carotid disease.

Deep Hemispheral Lesions. If the lesions are deep within the hemisphere, within the *internal capsule* or the *thalamus,* the face, arm, and leg are compromised equally (Fig. 10.1c). In these deep structures, nerves representing different parts of the contralateral body are confined within a small volume and are susceptible to the same lesions. Acute onset of transient numbness of half of the body suggests a TIA or a lacunar infarction in the posterior capsule or thalamus.

There is another distinction between the sensory loss resulting from cortical or from deep lesions. Lesions of the parietal cortex disturb complex discriminative modalities, such as two-point discrimination, but leave unaffected the primary modalities, such as pain, temperature, and vibration. Pain is not a prominent feature of cortical lesions. In contrast, *thalamic* lesions impair all primary modalities on the contralateral face, arm, and leg. There may be severe and persistent pain in all affected regions.

Brainstem Lesions. The hallmark of brainstem lesions is crossed findings— sensory findings on one side of the face and on the opposite arm and leg (Fig. 10.1d). Often a brainstem lesion is accompanied by cranial nerve, cerebellar, or motor findings. However, such accompanying signs are often minor. For example, sometimes only the crossed sensory findings alert the physician to a TIA or stroke involving the vertebral artery.

Spinal Cord Lesions. The distinctive features of spinal cord lesions are a sensory level: abnormal sensation below the level of the lesion, with normal sensation above. In complete lesions, there is also complete paralysis of limbs (as well as bowel and bladder) below the level of the lesion—giving rise to an inescapably obvious syndrome. Detection of partial lesions depends on finding a dissociated sensory loss in a distinctive pattern. Large-fiber sensory modalities, such as vibration, are mediated by fibers that traverse the spinal cord ipsilaterally, just as do motor fibers descending the cord. In contrast, small fibers carrying pain and temperature sensation transmit their signals to fibers crossing the middle of the spinal cord to ascend on the opposite side. These permit distinction of two partial spinal cord syndromes. Involvement of one side of the spinal cord results in a classic Brown-Séquard syndrome: impairment of vibratory sensation and motor function on one lower half and impairment of temperature sensation on the other (Fig. 10.1e). A central lesion, as in syringomyelia, involves only the crossing fibers subsuming small-fiber sensation in several dermatomes and spares the uncrossed long tracts in the posterior columns, which subsume large-fiber modalities of vibration and proprioception as well as the previously crossed small fibers. This gives rise to a capelike distribution of suspended sensory loss (Fig. 10.1f).

Functional (Hysterical) Numbness

The physician should suspect functional causes if there is a significant discrepancy between the pattern of a patient's symptoms and neuroanatomic or neurophysiologic realities. Some clues suggesting functional numbness include the following:

— abrupt change from profound abnormality to normal sensation without an intervening area of partial anesthesia. Such a pattern does not occur in structural lesions because there is always an area of overlap between adjacent nerve territories. Even if a nerve is totally interrupted, the border zone will be partially covered by its neighbor.
— impairment of sensation on one half of the body—hemisensory loss—accompanied by loss of olfaction, vision, and hearing on the same side of the body.
— impairment of joint and position sensation that is as severe proximally as it is distally. In neurologically impaired individuals, mild disease makes it difficult to detect small excursions at distal joints

of fingers and toes, while excursions of larger, more proximal joints such as wrist and ankle are still readily detected.

— profound sensory loss without signs of injury. A truly anesthetic limb deprived of protective reflexes is subject to bruises, cuts, and burns, which should be evident on physical examination even after only a few days.

— vibratory impairment on only one half of the frontal bone. The base of the nose and the forehead are each a single bone, which will vibrate as a unit after the application of a tuning fork. In a neurologically impaired individual, such transmitted vibration will be detected by the normal nerve on the other side of the face.

Nonneurological Sensory Impairment

Disorders that cause pain but are not associated with paresthesias or dysethesias usually emanate from joints, muscle, skin, subcutaneous tissues, or viscera. The pattern of such altered sensation does not correspond to one of the neurologic patterns described above. There may be local or even referred tenderness from deep palpation or manipulation, but the sensory examination will be normal.

Evaluation

History

A good history is more rewarding than a sensory examination. The physician should ask the patient to describe the sensory disturbance systematically: its onset, quality (e.g., sharp, dull, burning, aching, or prickling), and location. Does the spatial distribution of the pain suggest one of the neurologic patterns described above? Temporal features are also important: how long does it last; when is it better or worse? Precipitants as well as factors that aggravate or relieve the sensation can be valuable clues to diagnosis. These include posture, movement, food, stress, rest, and analgesics. The physician should record the severity of the pain on a scale of 0 to 10 as a way of gauging progression. Comparison of the patient's demeanor with the self-report of current severity can also be telling. Finally, the physician should inquire about associated symptoms, such as weakness, clumsiness, impaired sweating, unexpected burns, or other trauma. Only after such history taking is examination likely to be profitable.

Physical Examination

The sensory examination is the most difficult part of the exam, for both the patient and the physician. It should be performed only after the history and the rest of the general physical and neurologic examination have focused inquiry into discrimination among a few possibilities. For example, does the patient have a carpal tunnel syndrome or a cervical radiculopathy? Such focus is necessary because fatigue—on the part of both the examiner and the patient—precludes exhaustive testing of the body with all possible sensory modalities.

The purpose of the sensory examination is to determine not only the spatial pattern of disturbance, but also the nature of the impairment. A useful clinical distinction can be made between tests of elementary and discriminative sensory modalities. Elementary modalities include the so-called small-fiber modalities of pinprick pain and temperature and the large-fiber modalities of vibratory and position sensation. These are so named because of the caliber of the axons that transmit the relevant information from the periphery to the spinal cord. Light touch is an elementary modality mediated by both types of axon. Small-fiber sensation is conveniently assessed with a cool tuning fork or a pin. The physician must use a fresh pin for each patient, lest inadvertent puncture transmit infection. Vibratory sensation can be assessed by applying a tuning fork to bony prominences.

The discriminative modalities include two-point discrimination and stereognosis (the recognition of the shapes of unseen coins, keys, or erasers placed in the patient's hand), graphesthesia (identification of an unseen number traced on a patient's hand), and baresthesia (comparison of the weights of two similar objects). These perceptions require not only the higher integrative function of the parietal cortex, but also the integrity of the elementary modalities. Testing of cortically based discriminative modalities is meaningful only if peripheral nerves and spinal cord faithfully transmit the elementary information for processing by the cortex.

The patterns sought by the examiner are dictated by tentative conclusions drawn from the history and the preceding examination. In seeking one of the patterns described above, the physician should work from the area of decreased sensation to an area of normal sensation, a transition more easily detected by patients with neurologic impairment. If the pattern is complex, marking the borders with a pen can be useful. In patients with incomplete lesions, rarely will the pattern be an exact duplicate of a picture in a textbook. The object of the examination is to determine whether the pattern of loss is consistent with neurologic lesion and, if so, which of the lesions suggested by the previous history and physical examination is the most likely.

Finally, the examiner should attempt to elicit transient sensory symptoms by direct manipulation. If the physician suspects a cervical lesion, he or she should gently flex the patient's neck to test for the Lhermitte phenomenon, also known as barber's chair sign. When positive, the patient reports an electric shock shooting down the back or into the limbs. Although this was initially described as a sign of multiple sclerosis, it can result from any lesion affecting the posterior aspect of the spinal cord.

If the examiner suspects compression of a peripheral nerve, he or she should attempt to elicit Tinel's sign. Tapping on a damaged nerve may elicit tingling in its distal distribution. A positive sign indicates the presence of regenerating nerve fibers. These will be present if there is a lesion at or proximal to the site of percussion. In carpal tunnel syndrome, tapping over the flexor surface of the wrist will produce tingling in the distribution of the median nerve—the palmar surface of the hand, the thumb, and the adjacent fingers, sparing the pinky. Carpal tunnel syndrome may also be associated with Phalen's sign (tingling induced by complete flexion of the wrist for 30–60 seconds).

Primary Management

Primary management depends entirely on which disease entities remain reasonable possibilities after the initial clinical investigation is concluded. Management of patients with back pain and migraine is described in Chapters 11 and 12, respectively.

Compressive Neuropathies

In patients suspected of having compressive neuropathy, the suspected etiology, duration, and severity determine whether referral to a specialist is necessary. In most acute and subacute compressive neuropathies, the focus of treatment is the identification and removal of the extrinsic factor that produced the compression. The only other required intervention is the use of splints to avoid further compression. For example, if a previously healthy patient wakens from an anesthetic procedure with numbness, tingling, and weakness in an ulnar distribution, the most likely diagnosis is malposition of the limb during surgery. The patient should be reassured and a protective splint applied over the elbow to prevent further compression at the ulnar groove. Complete resolution of symptoms is expected within days to weeks. Only if improvement does not occur within this interval is referral to a neurologist necessary.

Even in patients with chronic compressive neuropathies, extrinsic exacerbating factors may be superimposed on intrinsically narrowed anatomic passageways. The physician should attempt to identify and reduce such exacerbating factors. Such measures include the use of splints, change of work habits to avoid recurrent compression, and a trial of antiinflammatory medications. Only if unacceptable symptoms persist after a month or two of such conservative treatment or if the cause of compression remains obscure should the physician refer for consideration of surgical decompression.

Radiculopathies

Management of lumbar radiculopathies resulting from disc or osteophytic disease is discussed in Chapter 11. The management of cervical radiculopathies resulting from analogous disease in the neck is similar. After high-velocity trauma or with long tract signs, such as hyperreflexia in the legs, or Lhermitte's sign of electrical shocks shooting down the back, there may be potentially lethal cervical instability or cord compression. In such cases, the physician should immobilize the patient's neck with sandbags or a hard collar and carefully transport the patient for radiography and neurosurgical evaluation. If, however, the signs and symptoms indicate root involvement without compromise to the cervical cord, evaluation can be done electively. Lateral cervical spine films should be taken in flexion and extension. If there is no significant instability, referral can be deferred unless a course of conservative management fails. Such conservative management includes analgesics, neck support, and a careful trial of cervical traction. Cervical traction can be performed at home with an apparatus available from most surgical supply houses or under the supervision of a physical therapist. It should be performed for 20 minutes daily, beginning with two pounds distraction and escalating as tolerated at two-day intervals by two-pound increments to a target of eight pounds. Traction should be discontinued immediately if symptoms worsen. Failure of symptoms to improve after several weeks should prompt referral to a specialist.

Functional or Unexplained Numbness

The demonstration of a nonphysiologic pattern of numbness suggests either malingering or hysteria but does not permit such a diagnosis. Both of these diagnoses require positive criteria. Above all, inability to identify the cause of persistent or recurring sensory complaints in the presence or absence of sensory findings on examination does not permit the presumption of a psychiatric diagnosis. As has been explained, diagnosis of sensory complaints is one of the most difficult exercises in neurology. Neurologic pathology can produce sensory symptoms in the absence of sensory or other confirmatory signs on examination. Frequently, nascent injuries give rise to partial patterns that may prove a difficult diagnostic exercise for even an experienced practitioner. Inability to make a diagnosis should be taken as simply that. Such patients should be followed with an open mind, watching for the evolution of a diagnostic pattern, with consultation if unexplainable symptoms persist.

Referral to a Specialist

For all central causes other than migraine, the physician should consider referral to a neurologist. If the history suggests a TIA, a stroke, or acute spinal cord or cauda equina compression, such referral should be made urgently

170 ■ VINAY CHAUDHRY

to an emergency room. A pattern suggestive of symmetric or multifocal peripheral neuropathy should also prompt such referral, as should all cases of persistent numbness in which the cause remains obscure.

Summary

The accurate diagnosis of only sensory complaints is a significant challenge to the physician. In the majority of cases, sensory complaints are part of a larger clinical constellation that can be recognized easily. Recognition of sensory symptoms indicative of significant underlying disease requires the identification of characteristic anatomic patterns. These patterns are most easily elicited from a careful history, which also reviews precipitating features and associated symptoms. Anatomic patterns suggested by the history and the remainder of the physical examination can often be confirmed by a strictly focused sensory examination. Absence of confirmatory signs on sensory testing should not prompt consideration of malingering or hysteria unless there is independent evidence to suggest such diagnoses.

ACKNOWLEDGMENT

The author thanks Dr. Neil Holland for permission to modify his drawings for use as Figure 10.1.

REFERENCES

Baringer, J. Richard. Herpes Zoster. In *Current Therapy in Neurologic Diseases,* 4th ed., edited by Richard T. Johnson and John W. Griffin, pp. 140–142. St. Louis: Mosby, 1993.

Plotkin, George M., and Dawson, David M. Entrapment Neuropathies. In *Current Therapy in Neurologic Diseases,* 5th ed., edited by Richard T. Johnson and John W. Griffin, pp. 377–380. St. Louis: Mosby, 1997.

Rosenbaum, Richard. Carpal Tunnel Syndrome. In *Current Therapy in Neurologic Diseases,* 5th ed., edited by Richard T. Johnson and John W. Griffin, pp. 374–376. St. Louis: Mosby, 1997.

Stewart, John D. *Focal Peripheral Neuropathies,* 3d ed. Philadelphia: Lippincott, Williams and Wilkins, 2000.

ELEVEN

Back Pain

John Dean Rybock, M.D.

Low back pain is an almost universal human experience. It is the second most common complaint encountered in medical practice. Some 15–20 percent of adults seek medical treatment for back pain each year, while another 30 percent may have episodic back pain that they treat themselves. Most of these patients can be well managed by the primary care physician. After exclusion of the presence of a few serious conditions that require immediate referral to a specialist, the role of the primary care physician is to minimize the period of disability and the risk of recurrence. This can be done without concern for a specific diagnosis. Only if there is a clear failure of initial treatment should there be an additional search for other specific diagnoses, such as herniated disc or spinal stenosis, that may require intervention by a specialist.

The Origin of Back Pain

The spinal column is a complex structure that must satisfy two competing functions: provide stable support for the body and allow a moderate range of motion. Each of the 25 bones in this stack is joined to its neighbors through three points of contact: the anteriorly placed intervertebral disc and a pair of facet joints posteriorly. Small muscles and ligaments interconnect the vertebrae. All of these structures are subjected to constant stresses, even from normal activities of daily living.

In an upright posture, these structures do not bear the body's weight evenly. The low back supports more weight than does the upper back and neck. Furthermore, both the neck and the low back develop inward curves, lordosis, so that the head can be balanced over the pelvis. However, virtually all the stresses of everyday life tend to collapse the spine anteriorly. These include the deposition of abdominal fat and the stresses imposed by lifting. Because of this delicate balance, relatively minor events can trigger strain or sprain of muscles, ligaments, intervertebral discs, or facet joints.

Initial Assessment

When a patient presents with acute low back pain, the primary care physician's initial goal is to determine whether there are any "red flags," signs or symptoms suggesting rare underlying diseases or injuries requiring urgent specialist treatment. These include fracture, infection, tumor, extraspinal disease with referred pain, and massive disc herniation (the cauda equina syndrome). Once these syndromes are excluded, the majority of patients will prove to have a self-limited syndrome and should initially be managed without further regard for specific diagnosis.

This initial distinction is provided by a focused history and physical examination. It is important to know whether the pain came on gradually or suddenly and whether there was any relation to trauma. If trauma is related to a motor vehicle accident or to injury at work, the details should be recorded. The location and quality of the pain are useful diagnostically, especially the presence of leg pain, particularly below the midthigh, and comparison of its intensity to the back pain. In addition, the severity of back pain, either by the patient's numerical ranking on a scale of 1 to 10 or by description of limitations on normal activities, must be recorded to provide a base from which to gauge progress. Symptoms suggesting neural compromise include weakness, numbness or abnormal sensations, or difficulties with bowel or bladder. The relationship of such symptoms and the pain to activity, position, and time of day is important.

In addition, the physician should ask the patient about systemic symptoms. Particularly relevant are unexplained weight loss; night sweats or fever; symptoms of abdominal, urologic, gynecologic, or vascular disease; and history of cancer, tuberculosis, sepsis, or use of steroids. It is also important to determine the psychosocial history, including work status, to know whether the physician should be concerned about secondary gain or similar complications.

The physician should examine the patient's back for focal tenderness, range of flexion and extension at the waist, and muscle tightness. Next, the physician should check for nerve root tension signs. With the patient supine, the examiner lifts the patient's straight leg, progressively flexing the hip. Exacerbation of radicular pain by this maneuver suggests impingement on a nerve root. The angle of the hip at which this occurs can be useful for monitoring progress. Neurologic examination of the legs and lower trunk includes examination of reflexes at the knee and ankle. Even mild degrees of weakness about the ankle can be detected by having the patient walk on heels and on toes.

Radiographic evaluation is not necessary during the initial evaluation unless the history or physical examination reveals red flags that warrant immediate intervention. Indeed, mild degrees of disc bulging or osteophytic spurring are common, even in asymptomatic individuals. Similar radiographic abnormalities in patients with an acute episode of back pain may not be directly related to the presenting complaint. Even when there is a direct relationship between a radiographically demonstrable anatomic lesion and an acute episode of back pain, its definition will not alter the acute management of the patient. For that reason, radiographic evaluation is sensibly deferred unless red flags are identified or the patient fails to recover after initial management.

Red Flags

After the initial assessment, the physician should consider whether there are red flags warning of an unusual problem that requires special management. Fracture should be suspected if the patient has fallen from a great height or been involved in a major collision. In otherwise healthy individuals, spinal fracture usually is accompanied by major injury to other organs. However, osteoporotic patients can suffer compression fractures, usually in the upper lumbar spine, even after minor trauma. If fracture is suspected, x-rays are indicated. Simple wedging without neurologic impairment can be managed with analgesics, a lumbosacral corset, and subsequent treatment of the bone disease. However, if there is malalignment or deformity, the physician should refer the patient to an orthopedic surgeon. Massive disc herniation after significant trauma can result in the cauda equina syndrome of pain, weakness, and numbness in both legs, as well as impairment of bowel and bladder function. Unlike typical lumbar disc herniation involving a single nerve root, this is a neurosurgical emergency.

Infection or tumor is a concern if there are signs or symptoms of systemic disease and continual pain not related to activity, usually worse at night. Infections usually develop in a single intervertebral disc space, visible on x-ray. Other destructive processes visible on x-ray are tumors, either intrinsic, such as myeloma, or metastatic from lung, breast, prostate, thyroid, or kidney. Extraspinal disease with referred pain most commonly results from renal calculi, enlargement of an aortic aneurysm, or pancreatitis.

Initial Treatment

In the absence of red flags, the patient requires reassurance and conservative management, not additional diagnostic testing. Even though many patients expect scans and x-rays, there is nothing on such studies that would change initial management. Even if there is a disc problem, it should first be given a chance to heal on its own. Indeed, false-positive findings on imaging can confuse the issue.

Education about risk factors for back stress is best begun at the initial visit. These risk factors include obesity, smoking, lack of regular exercise, and improper body mechanics. Activity should be limited for the first few days, with bed rest for disabling pain. However, prolonged bed rest leads to deconditioning and worsening of muscle spasm. Most back pain results from overcontraction of muscles. This can be avoided by a gradual increase of activity within a few days, with walking and stretching. A reasonable amount of activity will not aggravate the initial injury, even if a disc had been injured.

Medication should be given to those requiring relief of symptoms. Over-the-counter nonsteroidal antiinflammatory drugs are usually the best choice, with instructions to take the equivalent of prescription strength. Those who cannot tolerate these should take acetaminophen, up to four grams per day. Muscle relaxants are often prescribed but are rarely helpful. If nonsteroidal antiinflammatory drugs are inadequate, a short course of oxycodone or hydrocodone is usually more beneficial than benzodiazepines.

Physical therapy is best provided by the patient's own active stretching exercises and resumption of normal activity. Perhaps the most important role of the physical therapist is education in body mechanics and a back exercise program to begin when the acute episode resolves. Although there is some evidence that manipulation can marginally reduce the duration of acute episodes, no value of hot packs or ultrasound has been demonstrated.

The physician should follow the patient's progress by either office visits or telephone, with a brief survey at each encounter to ensure that red flags have not appeared. If there is no improvement after four to six weeks or there is persistent nerve root dysfunction with tension signs, the physician should consider further diagnostic workup, with a view to referral to a specialist.

Specific Diagnoses Requiring Later Referral to a Specialist

Apart from the diagnoses discussed in relation to red flags, the best-defined conditions requiring specialized treatment are persistent symptoms from disc herniation or lumbar stenosis. In addition, the diagnoses of degenerative disc disease and spondylosis may need clarification. Pursuit of these diagnoses is best deferred until after an adequate trial of conservative treatment. Lumbar disc herniation usually involves either the L5 or the S1 nerve root, both of which contribute to the sciatic nerve. The radiating pain of sciatica usually stops at the ankle, medially when L5 is compressed, laterally with S1. Sciatica is aggravated by activity or cough. Reclining with knees elevated is usually the most comfortable position.

Conservative treatment with proscription of activities that aggravate leg pain is preferable to strict bed rest and results in resolution of at least 70 percent of cases. Most cases will resolve in four to six weeks, but some take longer. If there is progressive improvement in symptoms, deficits, and nerve root tension signs, conservative treatment can be pursued safely until the problem resolves.

Should improvement fail, the physician should consider scanning in preparation for referral to a surgeon. Depending on local practice, it may be preferable to allow the specialist first to evaluate the patient and choose the appropriate imaging modality. Usually, high-resolution closed magnetic resonance imaging (MRI) is most appropriate. Open-air MRI, advocated by some for claustrophobic patients, usually fails to provide the necessary resolution, so its use should be discouraged. Elderly patients with sciatica resulting from bony spurs rather than soft discs are better imaged by computed tomographic (CT) scanning with two-dimensional (2D) and three-dimensional (3D) reconstructions. A small minority of patients require myelography with follow-up CT scanning. Nerve conduction studies and electromyography are usually not helpful. Root dysfunction detectable only by electrical studies but not clinically is unlikely to change treatment planning.

Lumbar stenosis is severe narrowing of the spine that results from slowly progressive degenerative changes in the spine. In addition to causing low back pain, it can result in a syndrome of "neurogenic claudication"—heaviness, numbness, and weakness in the legs after prolonged walking. Characteristically, the leg symptoms are relieved completely by one or two minutes of sitting. Symptoms are worse when the back is "straight" or extended. Flexing the back by leaning over a shopping cart can improve walking ability. In some cases, conservative management with an active exercise program (William's flexion exercises) can delay or prevent the need for surgery. However, an unacceptable degree of disability persisting after a good trial of exercise should prompt consideration of scanning and surgical referral.

Degenerative disc disease and lumbar spondylosis are best considered features of radiology reports rather than clinical diagnoses. These are a series of radiographic changes that occur in all individuals as a part of the aging process, even in individuals free of back pain. Lumbar spondylosis refers not only to degeneration of discs but also to accompanying changes in adjacent vertebral bodies, facet joints, and ligaments. In some individuals, bone spurs (osteophytes) can cause nerve root compression similar to that of a herniated disc or lumbar stenosis. Patients with the appropriate syndrome (radicular leg pain greater than back pain or neurogenic claudication) persisting after an adequate trial of conservative therapy are candidates for surgical evaluation.

Patients with predominately back pain in the absence of neurologic deficits, even with radiologic diagnoses of disc bulges or spondylosis, are generally not candidates for surgery. Such patients are best referred to a back specialist with nonsurgical alternatives—a physiatrist, neurosurgeon, or orthopedic surgeon providing a wider range of services such as neuroaugmentation, trigger point injections, and various nerve blocks.

Summary

Conservative management with rest, analgesics, and education is indicated for most cases of low back pain, whatever the etiology. The initial clinical evaluation not only provides a baseline assessment but also focuses on identification of "red flags" warning of unusual circumstances that warrant immediate referral for specialist treatment. Chief among these are metastatic tumor, vertebral infection, instability from high-velocity trauma, or severe bilateral neurologic deficit from central compression. Conservatively managed patients whose symptoms and signs show no significant improvement after an interval of four to six weeks should be investigated radiographically to search for surgically remediable lesions that could account for observed neurologic deficits. Surgical intervention for radiographically demonstrated abnormalities in the absence of an appropriate neurologic syndrome is usually not appropriate for the treatment of isolated back pain. Earlier surgical intervention of osteophytic or disc disease is unwarranted in most cases because symptoms tend to resolve spontaneously. After the resolution of acute symptoms, all patients need to institute a program of back care, diet, and exercise, either on direction of the physician or with the assistance of a physical therapist, to minimize the chances of recurrence.

REFERENCE

Rybock, John Dean. Low Back Pain and Lumbar Disc Herniation. In *Current Therapy in Neurologic Diseases*, 4th ed., edited by Richard T. Johnson and John W. Griffin, pp. 75–76. St. Louis: Mosby, 1993.

TWELVE

Headaches

David W. Buchholz, M.D.

Headaches are among the most common complaints that patients present to their physicians. In the large majority of cases, headaches do not herald significant underlying disease and can be managed by a primary practitioner. In a small minority of cases, headaches result from serious underlying diseases, some of which may require urgent evaluation and treatment. Other headaches, while not indicative of life-threatening illness, may indicate an unusual pathophysiology requiring treatment by an experienced practitioner.

The initial role of the primary care practitioner is to decide whether the history or physical examination contains danger signals indicating the need for referral for testing or to a specialist. Once such unusual cases are referred on, practitioners need a management plan for the vast majority of headache patients who will remain in their care. The initial step for these patients is the identification and avoidance of headache trigger factors. Headaches persisting after trigger factors are removed may require medication: interval treatment of infrequent headaches with analgesics and prophylactic treatment of frequent headaches.

When to Refer Headache Patients

When patients have the sudden onset of a uniquely severe headache, consider intracranial (especially subarachnoid) hemorrhage; these patients may be candidates for emergency evaluation including noncontrast computed tomographic (CT) scanning and lumbar puncture. Headache in the presence of fever and stiff neck may raise concern for meningitis. Other potential reasons for consideration of further evaluation include (1) headaches associated with persistent, unexplained neurological symptoms or signs (e.g., impaired mental status, focal sensorimotor deficits, or papilledema); (2) unprecedented, unexplained worsening of headaches; (3) headaches in patients with certain underlying problems (e.g., cancer, anticoagulation, human immunodeficiency virus [HIV]-AIDS); and (4) headaches that are refractory to appropriate migraine-preventive treatment. As a general rule, chronic headache patients without significant "red flags" do not require scanning or other tests beyond routine clinical evaluation.

Several specific headache disorders or illnesses associated with headaches or facial pain, such as cluster headache, giant cell (temporal) arteritis, idiopathic intracranial hypertension (pseudotumor cerebri), and trigeminal neuralgia, can be recognized clinically, as discussed below. Unless clinicians are comfortable with these entities, it is reasonable to refer patients suspected of having these diagnoses to a neurologist or some other appropriate consultant for further evaluation and management.

Cluster Headache

This primary, neurovascular headache disorder afflicts mostly men and is characterized by headache intervals (clusters) of a few months' duration separated by longer headache-free periods. A less common, chronic form of the disorder is without headache-free periods. During a headache interval, the individual has one to several episodes per day of excruciating, unilateral, periorbital pain—consistently on the same side during an interval—lasting one-half to one hour or so. Episodes often arise from sleep. There may be accompanying ipsilateral redness and tearing of the eye, ptosis, and nasal congestion. People with cluster headaches tend to be highly agitated during their headaches. Alcohol is an immediate trigger for most patients during headache intervals (but not in headache-free periods).

Acute treatment of cluster headache involves either inhalation of 100 percent oxygen or injection of sumatriptan. Preventive treatment—initiated at the onset of a headache interval and continued for its usual duration—includes either verapamil (in dosages ranging from 240 to 960 mg qd), divalproex (up to 750–1,000 mg qd), prednisone (tapering from 60–80 mg qd), or methysergide (up to 4 mg tid). Lithium is an option for chronic cluster headache.

Giant Cell (Temporal) Arteritis

Immune-mediated inflammation of the temporal and other extracranial arteries produces headache and temporal artery tenderness, often accompanied by palpable abnormalities in the temporal arteries. Suspect this disorder in elderly persons, especially those with associated systemic symptoms of polymyalgia rheumatica (myalgias, fatigue, malaise, and anorexia). The erythrocyte sedimentation rate usually (but not always) is markedly elevated, but prompt temporal artery biopsy should be obtained for diagnosis. Urgent corticosteroid therapy is indicated, lest delayed treatment result in ocular ischemia and permanent visual loss.

Idiopathic Intracranial Hypertension (Pseudotumor Cerebri)

This condition, which results in increased intracranial pressure and consequent headaches and visual disturbances, should be considered especially in young, obese women and is almost always associated with papilledema. After a brain CT or magnetic resonance imaging (MRI) scan (to rule out a mass lesion or hydrocephalus), the diagnosis is confirmed by lumbar puncture and careful cerebrospinal fluid pressure measurement—with the patient as relaxed as possible and with legs extended, to avoid artifactually elevated pressure due to the Valsalva effect. Treatment is indicated not only to relieve headaches but also to prevent permanent optic nerve damage, and options include multiple lumbar punctures, acetazolamide, corticosteroids, lumboperitoneal shunting, and fenestration of the optic nerve sheath.

Trigeminal Neuralgia

Recurrent paroxysms of lightning-like, electrical shock-type pain across one side of the face—often triggered by light touch—characterize this disorder. It is most common among the elderly, in whom it is thought to be due to a tortuous artery near the brainstem causing irritation of the trigeminal nerve. Nonetheless, it may occur at any age, and scanning should be considered to rule out a tumor or aneurysm along the pathway of the nerve.

Medications such as carbamazepine, phenytoin, or baclofen are usually effective, but refractory cases may require glycerol injection or microvascular decompression (via posterior fossa craniotomy).

The Diagnosis and Treatment of Chronic Headaches

Clinicians are often frustrated by patients who continue to complain of chronic headaches despite extensive efforts at diagnosis and treatment. This frustration fosters a tendency to regard these "failed" headache patients as having a psychogenic problem or being complainers or drug seekers. In truth, it is clinicians, not patients, who in most cases are responsible for the failure of headache treatment because the conventional wisdom about headache diagnosis and treatment, to which most clinicians adhere, is faulty.

A better way of looking at chronic headaches enables clinicians to guide patients—even patients for whom treatment has failed—to effective headache control. The approach is simple but not always easy, especially at the start. The first step is to understand that the mechanism of migraine is responsible for the vast majority of headaches, including headaches of all types. The next step is migraine-preventive treatment, which begins with elimination of avoidable trigger factors (mainly certain dietary items and medications) and may or may not require preventive medication. The third step is *judicious* use of analgesic medication in appropriate patients under the right circumstances. The final step is to recognize when headaches are "rebounding" from overuse of analgesic medication—because rebounding not only generates increased headaches but also blocks responsiveness to migraine-preventive treatment—and to eliminate rebounding, which requires elimination of the responsible analgesics.

Each of these steps is discussed in detail below. The ultimate goal of this approach to chronic headaches is not to eradicate headaches. The goal is to guide patients from a situation in which their headaches and headache medications have control over them to a situation in which they have control over their headaches and headache treatment. Instead of the management of chronic headaches being frustrating for both patients and clinicians, this simple approach to the problem is mutually gratifying.

The Mechanism and Spectrum of Migraine

Too often the term *migraine* is used to denote a specific type of headache— that is, a severe, unilateral, throbbing headache lasting for a few hours to a few days, accompanied by nausea and photophobia, and sometimes associated with visual disturbances. This definition of migraine is narrow and misleading. A better way to think of migraine is as a mechanism that generates a broad spectrum of headaches, at the far end of which lies the type of headaches described above—that is, those that are conventionally labeled migraines. Along this spectrum lie all types of headaches, including mild to moderate, nonspecific headaches, unaccompanied by other symptoms, that are usually mislabeled as "tension," "stress," or "sinus" headaches. Of course, when headaches are mislabeled and misunderstood as to their underlying mechanism, treatment is likely to be misdirected and ineffective, and frustration will ensue.

The details of the mechanism of migraine are largely lacking, but a conceptual model can be offered. Even if this model is overly simplistic, it nonetheless provides clinicians and patients a reasonable handle to grasp in the process of gaining control over headaches. In the brain is a control center that governs the mechanism of migraine. The location of the migraine control center is speculative, but the hypothalamus is a reasonable candidate. When the control center is activated, so is the mechanism, and the level of activation in the control center determines the level of activity of the mechanism overall. In explaining this to patients, it is useful to use the analogy of a radio control knob that clicks on and then can be adjusted so as to turn the volume up or down. When the migraine control center is turned up all the way, patients are likely to experience severe headaches that are recognized as migraines, but when the mechanism is only partially activated, the result is milder, nonspecific headaches that are likely to be regarded as something else, such as tension headaches.

Two things determine whether the migraine control center is activated and, if so, to what degree. One is its threshold of activation. This is largely hereditary, such that headache-prone individuals, who tend to come from headache-prone families, have low thresholds on a genetic basis. Matched against the threshold of activation is a stack of trigger factor input derived from many different sources including hormones, stress, dietary items, barometric pressure changes, and sleep disturbances. If the total level of trigger factors stays below the threshold, the migraine control center and the mechanism it governs are inactive. If the trigger factor level crosses the threshold, the mechanism is turned on, and the higher the trigger factor level climbs above the threshold, the more fully activated the mechanism becomes.

Beyond its control center the mechanism of migraine involves a complicated cascade of events in various parts of the brain and brainstem, mediated by multiple neurotransmitters. The mechanism of migraine can be blunted by drugs that stimulate serotonin receptors, block dopamine receptors, and inhibit prostaglandin synthesis, implying that at least these (and probably other) chemical mediators play roles.

The culmination of this cascade of events in the brain and brainstem is activation of a migraine generator in the brainstem, probably involving the trigeminal nucleus caudalis. Efferent trigeminal nerve fibers carry impulses that lead to release of neuropeptides (such as substance P and calcitonin gene-related peptide) from perivascular nerve endings. These neuropeptides produce extracerebral vasodilation and vascular inflammation in the meninges and other tissues around the head. Vasodilation and vascular inflammation produce discomfort, and the degree, duration, and localization of discomfort vary widely depending on the degree, duration, and localization of these neurovascular changes, which in turn depend on the level of activation of the mechanism of migraine that gives rise to them.

Not only is the term *migraine* narrow and misleading in its common usage, but also even the term *headache* is narrow and misleading. Discomfort generated by the mechanism of migraine may be felt anywhere in or around the face, head, or neck. Patients may experience discomfort that they describe using many words other than *ache,* and their discomfort may be felt unilaterally or bilaterally in the eyes, sinuses, teeth, jaw, ears, scalp, neck, or "shoulders" (trapezius muscle regions) rather than in the "head." Patients commonly distinguish multiple types of discomfort that they often call by different names—for example, migraines, sinus headaches, and tension headaches—that feel different from each other and may occur independently, yet they all stem from the same source (the mechanism of migraine) activated to varying degrees and expressing itself in a variety of ways. As headache patients go through life, their manifestations of migraine are liable to change.

The mechanism of migraine gives rise not only to discomfort in and around the head. It also results in autonomic disturbances and a wide array of neurologic symptoms. These other symptoms of migraine may or may not be associated with discomfort. Autonomic symptoms—including nausea, vomiting, diarrhea, constipation, pallor, flushing, sweating, and fever—probably reflect hypothalamic involvement in the mechanism of migraine.

The neurologic symptoms of migraine vary in duration from seconds to hours or more and include a variety of visual disturbances (blurring, spots, flashing lights), vestibular symptoms (dizziness, disequilibrium, vertigo), auditory changes (tinnitus, muffled hearing), sensory disturbances (hemifacial or migratory hemibody tingling), and cognitive dysfunction (difficulty concentrating, transient global amnesia). There is controversy as to the origin of these symptoms. The most common explanations are intracranial vasospasm, spreading depression of neuronal function, or some process combining these two phenomena.

Mythical Causes of Headaches

Two myths, in particular, pervade headache diagnosis. The first is that of tension or stress headaches. Many clinicians were taught (and still believe) that mild to moderate, nonspecific headaches—the vast majority of headaches—are caused by emotional or psychological problems leading to excessive contraction of muscles around the head and neck, in turn producing pain. Electromyographic studies, however, have failed to show any consistent relationship between excessive contraction of head and neck muscles and the types of headaches that are labeled as tension or stress headaches. Although this hypothesis has come to be rejected by most headache specialists, it remains part of conventional wisdom. Consequently, misdiagnosis of the nature of headaches leads to misguided (and ultimately failed) treatment and creates frustration.

The second major myth of headache diagnosis is sinus headaches. Although it is true that acute infective sinusitis can produce retrofacial pain, it is likely to be accompanied by other symptoms of infection including purulent discharge and fever. Chronic, recurrent retrofacial pain and congestion, unaccompanied by specific symptoms of infection, too often are attributed inappropriately to sinus infection, allergies, or anatomic abnormalities (e.g., polyps, mucosal thickening, or nasal septal deviation) without clear-cut evidence of any relationship between these considerations and the patients' pain complaints and despite persistent complaints in the face of extensive treatment with antihistamines, decongestants, topical steroids, antibiotics, allergy shots, and even sinus surgery.

The mechanism of migraine has a predilection for causing vasodilation and vascular inflammation in the richly vascular muscosa lining the nose and sinuses. This results in retrofacial pain and congestion, but these symptoms are usually attributed to something other than migraine, as discussed above. Ironically, the diagnosis of vasomotor rhinosinusitis is an apt description of the process, but conventional wisdom has not linked this diagnosis with migraine because of the tendency to fixate on migraine as a type of headache rather than to recognize it as a mechanism generating vasomotor changes and inflammation that can be perceived in many different ways.

Other factors have conspired to obscure recognition of migraine causing sinus symptoms. Nonspecific findings of imaging studies, such as mucosal thickening on x-rays or CT scans or increased signal intensity on MRI scans, are routinely reported to represent "sinusitis," implying an infective process. Clinicians are more likely to respond reflexively by prescribing antibiotics and decongestants rather than by considering that the findings may represent migrainous mucosal engorgement. Confusion also stems from the fact that patients with migraine causing sinus symptoms may seem to respond to therapy, even when it is misdirected, because decongestants are vasoconstrictors that may temporarily reverse migrainous mucosal vasodilation, thereby reinforcing the misdiagnosis of what is really a migraine problem as an infection or a response to allergies. Further complicating the recognition of migraine is the potential for migrainous mucosal engorgement to block sinus drainage and thereby lead to secondary bacterial infection, an epiphenomenon that may be misconstrued as the underlying problem.

There are many other, less common myths—or, at least, misguided tendencies—in headache diagnosis. Too often headaches are attributed to routine degeneration of the cervical spine shown on imaging studies. When patients are symptomatic from cervical spine disease, it is usually because of spinal nerve root compression causing radiating upper extremity symptoms, not neck pain or headaches. Temporomandibular (TM) joint dysfunction may cause problems with jaw opening and local pain but is unlikely to be the source of pain away from the TM joints.

The Elimination of Trigger Factors

The first step in preventive treatment of migraine is to try to keep the total level of trigger factors below the threshold of activation. This is accomplished by eliminating trigger factors that are avoidable—recognizing that, for practical purposes, many important trigger factors cannot be avoided, including stress, hormones, and barometric pressure changes. This fact makes it all the more important to focus on the *avoidable* trigger factors. For the most part avoidable trigger factors are things that patients put in their mouths and swallow: certain dietary items (Table 12.1) and medications (Table 12.2).

Patients tend to recognize few if any of their dietary trigger factors, and, to comply with a migraine-preventive diet that eliminates these potential factors, they must understand why they have not figured this out for themselves. The first reason is that dietary trigger factors can act on a delayed basis, 24 hours or more after consumption. Second, no individual dietary item determines whether a headache will occur or how severe it will be. Headache activity is determined by the total sum of trigger factor input—

Table 12.1. Dietary Trigger Factors of Migraine

Item	Comment
Caffeine	Coffee, tea, iced tea, and cola; even decaffeinated coffee and tea may be a problem.
Chocolate	
Cheese	Avoid all cheeses except American, cream, and cottage cheese. Avoid cheese-containing foods, such as pizza.
Monosodium glutamate	Chinese restaurant food, many snack foods and prepared foods, Accent and other seasoning products; MSG may be labeled as hydrolyzed vegetable/soy/plant protein, natural flavorings, yeast extract, Kombu, broth, stock, and others; *read labels.*
Yogurt and sour cream	
Nuts	Including peanut butter
Processed meats	Those that are aged, canned, cured, marinated, or tenderized or that contain nitrates or nitrites, including hot dogs, sausage, bacon, salami, and bologna
Alcohol and vinegar	Especially red wine, champagne, and dark or heavy drinks; vodka is best tolerated; white vinegar is OK.
Citrus fruits and juices	Oranges, grapefruits, lemons, limes, and pineapples and their juices; vitamin C and citric acid are OK.
Certain other fruits	Bananas, raisins, red plums, canned figs, and avocados
Certain vegetables	Lima, fava, and navy beans; pea pods; sauerkraut; and onions
Certain bread products	Yeast-risen bread products less than one day old—as from a bakery, doughnut shop, or home
Aspartame (Nutrasweet)	

derived from many different sources, both dietary and nondietary—in relation to the threshold of activation. One day, the consumption of a dietary item may push the trigger factor level above the threshold, thereby triggering a headache; the next day, however, starting with a lower level of trigger factors, consumption of the same dietary item may not raise the trigger factor level past the threshold, and a headache will not occur. Patients tend to misinterpret such experiences as indicating that the dietary item in question does not contribute to their headaches because it doesn't always cause a headache, not realizing that the dietary item always contributes to the likelihood of a headache, even though it does not always cause a headache.

Another reason for confusion about dietary items is the paradoxical effect of those containing caffeine. In the short run, caffeine, being a vasoconstrictor, may help to relieve a headache. However, decreased caffeine intake may result in withdrawal headaches because caffeine-induced vasoconstriction is followed by rebound vasodilation. In the long run, therefore, caffeine promotes headaches and must be avoided. Advise patients that

Table 12.2. Medication Trigger Factors

Medication	Example
Hormones	Birth control pills
	Hormone replacement therapy
Adrenaline-like drugs, stimulants, and diet pills	Bronchodilators
	Over-the-counter stimulants
	Methylphenidate (Ritalin)
	Dextroamphetamine sulfate (Dexedrine)
	Over-the-counter diet pills
	Prescription diet pills
Vasodilators	Nitrates for heart disease
	Sildenafil citrate (Viagra)

withdrawal from caffeine, although the right thing to do, may be associated with increased headaches for up to a few weeks.

The wisest way to use a migraine-preventive diet is to be as strict as possible until satisfactory headache control is achieved (which may require additional preventive measures), after which dietary items can be added back one at a time to see what items (and what quantities of these items) can be tolerated without losing headache control. Dietary restriction may or may not be sufficient to achieve satisfactory headache control (i.e., to keep the total trigger factor level below the threshold of activation most of the time). When dietary restriction is not sufficient and other steps need to be taken (such as adding preventive medication), the diet is nonetheless *necessary* for additional steps to be effective.

Medications can also act as trigger factors for the mechanism of migraine (see Table 12.2), but sometimes it is not in the best overall interest of patients to eliminate these medications because they may be providing some greater benefit. As with potential dietary trigger factors, elimination of these medications may or may not be sufficient to achieve headache control but should be considered as part of a multifaceted preventive treatment program. Also, like dietary trigger factors, these medications may be reintroduced to see whether the patient can tolerate them, *after* headache control has been achieved.

The Proper Use of Preventive Medication

For a migraine-preventive medication to work, it must be used in the proper setting. The proper setting includes elimination of rebounding and of avoidable trigger factors. If these steps have been taken and a patient continues to have unsatisfactory headache severity and frequency, then preventive medication is an appropriate next step.

Preventive medication options are listed in Table 12.3. The initial dosage should be low to avoid side effects, and dosage should be steadily increased over one to two months until the patient achieves satisfactory headache control, has intolerable side effects that cannot be circumvented, or is taking the maximal allowable dosage. If one preventive medication is ineffective despite maximal tolerable/allowable dosage, the next option should be substituted in its place. If a preventive medication is partially effective, but the dosage cannot be raised further, it is reasonable to leave that medication in place and add a second preventive medication to it. If headache control is achieved with the second medication, the first medication can be tapered to determine whether it is needed. Most headaches requiring preventive medication can be controlled with a single agent, but some patients benefit from a combination of two or even three, each added one at a time.

Too often preventive medications that would have worked well if given a fair trial are rejected because of side effects that could have been circumvented. For example, excessive morning sedation after the initiation of a tricyclic antidepressant often improves within a few days to weeks or can be

Table 12.3. Migraine-Preventive Medications

Medication	Initial Dosage	Maximal Dosage
Tricyclic antidepressants		
Nortriptyline or amitriptyline	10–25 mg hs	100–200 mg hs
Calcium channel blockers		
Verapamil or diltiazem	120 mg qd or bid	240 mg bid
Divalproex sodium	125–250 mg hs	1,000–1,500 mg bid
Beta blockers		
Nadalol	20 mg qd	80 mg bid
Propranolol	40 mg qd	160 mg bid
Cyproheptadine	2–4 mg hs	8 mg tid

reduced either by lowering the dosage (and raising it more gradually) or by taking the medication earlier in the evening. Constipation from tricyclic antidepressants or verapamil can usually be managed with routine measures such as fiber supplementation, or verapamil can be switched to diltiazem. Beta blockers and calcium channel blockers should not be reduced or eliminated simply because of relative bradycardia or hypotension without symptoms or special cause for concern.

In many patients, preventive medications can eventually be reduced or eliminated without sacrificing headache control because patients' headache tendencies may subside over time for reasons that may or may not be identifiable. After several months or more of satisfactory headache control, it is reasonable to try lowering the dosage of preventive medication, seeing what happens, and making further dosage adjustments accordingly.

The Appropriate Use of Analgesics

Mild to moderate headaches are appropriately treated with plain aspirin, acetaminophen, or an antiinflammatory agent. These medications probably do not cause rebounding and therefore could be used as often as several times per week without fear of that complication, but usage of any analgesic so frequently indicates that preventive treatment should be undertaken or upgraded. Antiinflammatory agents are most likely to be effective if they are taken early and at relatively high dosage (e.g., 600–800 mg of ibuprofen or 440–660 mg of naproxen sodium).

Simple analgesics and antiinflammatories are unlikely to work for severe headaches. It is reasonable to treat infrequent severe headaches with a prescription analgesic, and triptans, from which there are a number to choose, are generally the best option as long as there is no contraindication, such as probable coronary artery disease. The problems with using triptans or other prescription analgesics too often—namely, decreased compliance with preventive treatment and the development of rebounding—are discussed below.

The Pitfalls of Rebounding

Rebounding refers to the increased headache tendency that occurs when an analgesic taken for relief of acute headache wears off. If certain remedies for acute headache are overused—more than once per week—the underlying headache tendency grows. Rebounding is usually not apparent in the short run (i.e., from dose to dose of analgesics) but is played out in the long run, over months and years. Patients gradually experience more frequent and severe headaches, as a result of which they consume more and more analgesics, usually not recognizing the vicious cycle taking place.

Many analgesics can lead to rebounding:

— Caffeine-containing analgesics
— Butalbital compounds
— Decongestants
— Isometheptene compounds
— Ergotamines
— Triptans
— Opioids

Plain aspirin, acetaminophen, and nonsteroidal antiinflammatory drugs (NSAIDs) probably do not produce rebounding. The mechanism of rebounding is unclear, but the properties of the medications associated with rebounding suggest at least two possibilities. Most of these medications are vasoconstrictors that may promote rebound vasodilation. In the case of opioids, the mechanism of rebounding may be related to changes in receptor sensitivity brought about by repeated binding of receptors by these medications.

The negative effect of rebounding is not just that it causes headaches to spin further out of control. Even worse, rebounding blocks responsiveness to migraine-preventive treatment. Despite best efforts to put on the brakes using migraine-preventive treatment, headaches will be driven forward—more and more out of control—by rebounding, and the brakes will fail. Rebounding must be eliminated for migraine-preventive treatment to become effective.

The ideal solution to rebounding is to avoid it in the first place. Chronic headache patients should be guided toward preventive treatment. Patients with *frequent* severe headaches should not be given rescue therapy in the form of prescription analgesics. These medications are appropriate for patients with *infrequent* severe headaches: those whose headaches are infrequent by nature or who have achieved reasonable headache control with preventive treatment but still have infrequent severe breakthrough headaches.

There are two problems with prescribing analgesics to patients with frequent severe headaches. First, availability of these medications is likely to undermine compliance with preventive treatment. Preventive treatment, when done properly, is highly effective in controlling headaches, but it takes time and effort. Preventive treatment, unlike rescue therapy, is not immediately gratifying. Once preventive treatment is established and effective, the reward of headache control reinforces preventive treatment and promotes continued compliance. In its early stages, however, preventive treatment is likely to be seen as hard work with no benefit, and patients are likely to veer off course if a handy detour—rescue therapy—is available, rather than staying on the right track with preventive treatment. The second problem with prescribing analgesics to patients with frequent severe headaches is that they probably will develop rebounding and, consequently, increased headaches, and it is difficult for them to acknowledge or address this problem once they have become dependent on analgesics.

Even when patients who are rebounding acknowledge the problem and are willing to address it, elimination of the problem—that is, stopping the medication(s) involved—is difficult. Patients are not only without their usual crutch to lean on but also are likely to experience increased headaches for a few weeks as a result of withdrawal. Except in certain cases involving opioids that need to be tapered, a "cold turkey" approach is best because it is definitive; too often, tapering never reaches its intended conclusion.

Some patients may need to be hospitalized for support during withdrawal, but this itself is a sort of rescue therapy, and there is the risk that patients who are hospitalized for withdrawal will be prescribed some other acute headache remedy to keep them quiet, thereby perpetuating the prob-

Table 12.4. Reasons for Treatment Failure

Your headache diagnosis is wrong.
You are relying too much on quick fixes and crisis management.
Your headache patient is rebounding.
Your patient is not avoiding headache trigger factors.
You are not prescribing preventive medications properly.
Your headache patient or you have unrealistic goals.
Your headache patient has a hidden agenda.
Your headache patient has coexistent psychological problems.
Your patient has an intractable headache problem.
Your headache patient does not understand the headache problem or its solution.

NOTE: This list was developed in conjunction with Stephen G. Reich, M.D.

lem of rebounding but under a different name. Preventive therapy can be instituted at the same time that patients are eliminating the medication(s) from which they are rebounding, but it is unlikely that preventive treatment will make elimination of rebounding easy, and patients should not expect preventive treatment to become effective until weeks to months after rebounding has been eliminated.

Why Headache Treatment Fails

Table 12.4 lists 10 reasons why chronic headaches fail to respond to treatment. The first five reasons have been discussed in detail. When patients report unsatisfactory results despite proper attention to these issues, consider the presence of a hidden agenda (e.g., litigation or disability) or other emotional or psychological problems (e.g., depression or family issues) that may be impeding either patients' responses to treatment or their reporting of favorable responses.

The importance of the last item on the list—that is, patients not understanding their headache problem and its solution—cannot be overemphasized. Although it takes time, it is essential that headache patients be educated as to the nature of their problem (i.e., the mechanism of migraine and, if appropriate, rebounding) and the importance of eliminating avoidable trigger factors. For instance, if patients don't receive an explanation as to why they have not recognized all of their dietary trigger factors on their own, they are unlikely to comply with the diet. In the long run, taking time to educate patients fully about their headache problem and its solution not only saves patients from suffering from headaches but also saves clinicians from spending much more time being interrupted for crisis management of headaches.

Summary

The vast majority of patients with chronic headaches suffer from the mechanism of migraine, and many are rebounding because of dependence on analgesics. To begin with, they must stop rebounding. Then, control of their migraine problem can be achieved by a strict preventive approach starting with elimination of avoidable trigger factors—especially certain dietary items and medications—and, if necessary, moving on to preventive medication. When appropriate preventive treatment fails to control headaches, considerations should be given to confounding hidden agendas and other emotional and psychological problems. Uncommonly, patients have headaches due to some problem other than migraine, but these patients almost always present with red flags that signify the need for specialized evaluation.

REFERENCES

Buchholz, D. W., and Reich, S. G. The Menagerie of Migraine. *Seminars in Neurology* 16 (1996): 83–93.
Moskowitz, M. A. Neurogenic Inflammation in the Pathophysiology and Treatment of Migraine. *Neurology* 43, suppl. 3 (1993): 16–20.
Olesen, J. The Ischemic Hypotheses of Migraine. *Archives of Neurology* 44 (1987): 321–322.
Raskin, N. H. *Headache,* 2d ed. New York: Churchill Livingstone, 1988.
Sacks, O. W. *Migraine.* Berkeley and Los Angeles: University of California Press, 1992.
Welch, K. M. Migraine: A Biobehavioral Disorder. *Archives of Neurology* 44 (1987): 323–327.

THIRTEEN

Dizzy Spells

Peter W. Kaplan, M.B., B.S., F.R.C.P.

Dizzy spells—brief alterations of consciousness, movement, or sensation—are frequent complaints. They are often alarming, impairing the ability of the patient or witness to recall exact features or chronology. Circumstances surrounding the event are often forgotten and need to be ferreted out; the time course of the event often assumes a larger scale: seconds become minutes, and minutes become tens of minutes. And if there is a fall, witnesses may be able to think of only "heart attack," "death," or "stroke" and be unable to observe signal features such as skin color, eye position, fluttering of the eyelids, or preceding staring or automatisms. This poses a special diagnostic challenge to the physician, who must rely on the description of an event that he or she has not witnessed, to make initial management decisions. The role of the primary care physician is to determine whether the description of the dizzy spell suggests an underlying cause requiring specialist treatment, further workup, or simple reassurance. Often the focus of the initial inquiry is to determine whether the patient is reporting a seizure.

Types of Dizzy Spells

Dizzy spells are events with an identifiable onset, subjective manifestations, and sometimes objective manifestations that can be seen by others. The patient may complain "I feel off," "off balance," "dizzy," or "lightheaded" or may include descriptions of perceptual distortions. Bystanders may observe alterations in behavior, cognition, or awareness. Many of the sensations are poorly described. It therefore requires a persistent examiner, using a language familiar to the patient, to establish what is meant by particular terms and then to use examples to enlarge the patient's (or witness's) ability to describe the dizzy spell. Clinicians often find themselves working with individual complaints from which a diagnosis must be made, but usually individual symptoms are shared by many diagnoses.

It is important to determine whether the patient and the physician are using these terms in the same way. *Dizziness* means different things to different people. It may mean unsteadiness, lightheadedness, imbalance, malaise, generalized weakness, a feeling of impending or actual loss of consciousness, or a perception of movement or rotation. A more specific explanation of the symptom is needed. More specific terms include *vertigo, lightheadedness,* and *presyncope.*

Vertigo can be used to identify the feeling of spinning, movement, or tilting in space, usually when a person is in the horizontal plane or when there are identifiable changes in position. It commonly suggests problems of the inner ear or the vestibular connections in the brainstem. Somewhat similar is the term *lightheadedness,* by which the patient may mean a sensation of pressure, airiness, tightness, fullness, or swaying. There may be a perception of floating, of "I was about to faint," or dimming of vision while the subject remains conscious. *Presyncope* describes a sensation of near fainting, very similar to lightheadedness but closer to what one would expect "before a faint." This may involve the perception (shortly after rising from a lying or sitting position) of ringing in the ears, a feeling of distance or remoteness, a drained feeling, or a graying out of vision. Many of these entities have overlapping features, and all at some point may be associated with nausea, vomiting, pallor, an unsteady gait, or a fast heart rate.

Frequent causes of typical dizzy spells are the following:

— Presyncope
— Syncope
— Inner ear problems; benign paroxysmal positional vertigo
— Anxiety
— Seizures
— Transient ischemic attacks
— Migraine

Table 13.1. Differentiating Features among Common Types of Dizzy Spells

Feature	Syncope	Tonic-Clonic Seizures	Psychogenic "Seizures"	Complex Partial Seizures	Migraine Variant	Vestibular Problems	Anterior Cerebral TIA	Posterior Cerebral TIA	Toxic/Metabolic (encephalopathy)
Premonitory symptoms	Sweating, light-headedness, graying of vision	Sometimes an aura (with partial onset only)	Varied	Sometimes an aura	Malaise, visual symptoms	None	None	None	Usually
Onset	Gradual	Sudden	Variable	Sudden	Gradual	Sudden	Sudden	Sudden	Yes but poorly identifiable
Stereotypy	Yes	Yes	Variable	Yes	Yes	Yes	Yes (if one vascular territory)	Yes (if one vascular territory)	Variable
Posture at onset	Usually standing	Any	Any	Any	Any	A particular position	Any	Any	Gradual: 30 min to hours
Progression and duration	Brief	Usually brief	Often prolonged	Brief	Prolonged	Prolonged	Sudden; variable but may last up to 24 hr	Sudden; variable but may last up to 24 hr	Very gradual
Postevent condition	Normal	Confusion, lethargy	Normal	Confusion	Normal	Normal	Normal	Normal	Normal
Convulsive movements	Occasionally	Common	Common	None	Never	Never	None	None	None
Injury with spell	Uncommon	Common	Rare	Uncommon	Never	Rare	Occasionally	Occasionally	Rarely
Incontinence	Rarely	Common	Rare	Rare	Never	Never	Rarely	Rarely	Rarely
Other features	Palpitations, slumping to the ground, stress before event	Sleep afterward, labored breathing	Waxing and waning, pelvic thrusting, thrashing about	Staring, lip-smacking, fidgeting, vocalizations	Headache, nausea, vomiting	Tinnitus, ear pain, ear infection	Lateralized visual loss, aphasia, lateralized extensive weakness or numbness	Diplopia, perioral numbness, loss of consciousness	Associated by history with drugs or medications

—Hypoglycemia

—Alcohol

—Recreational or prescription drugs

—Delirium

—Panic attacks and hyperventilation

—Hysteria, conversion disorders, malingering

—Sleep disorders

Often the diagnostic challenge is to determine whether the patient may have had a seizure or transient ischemic attack (TIA)—conditions requiring neurologic investigation—or some other condition, including other types of neurologic problems, such as migraine or narcolepsy, otolaryngologic problems from the inner ear, and psychiatric problems such as anxiety.

Diagnoses are usually based on the constellation of symptoms offered by the patient and signs described by witnesses. Because patients come to the physician with signs and symptoms and not discrete diagnoses, this chapter outlines some of the typical constellations of clinical features and clinical conditions. An abbreviated list comparing particular clinical features of several types of dizzy spells is provided in Table 13.1.

Seizures

Seizures are a common cause of dizzy spells, the result of paroxysmal disorganized electrical activity in the cerbral cortex. The varying spread and degree of epileptic discharge results in a wide spectrum of clinical expression. Clinical features may, therefore, vary from the entirely subjective (e.g., an "aura"—perhaps a bad smell—or fear [simple partial seizure]) to the objective (staring, fidgeting, and loss of consciousness of which the patient is not aware). If the abnormal electrical discharge involves both hemispheres, there is usually loss of consciousness.

Tonic-Clonic Seizures

Generalized tonic-clonic seizures rarely present diagnostic challenges. They are usually unprovoked and sudden in onset. There is loss of consciousness and a tonic stiffening of jaw and limbs, followed by a period of sustained clonic repetitive jerking that lasts about a minute. Afterward, the limbs relax and the patient regains consciousness over several minutes, initially confused and disoriented. After regaining consciousness, the patient may experience a mild headache and then fall asleep for a brief period. Because of the violence of the muscle contractions, there is often incontinence of bladder, sore muscles, and a bitten lip. Generalized tonic-clonic seizures must be differentiated from convulsive syncope, in which there may be three to four clonic jerks as consciousness is lost but no incontinence or confusion after consciousness is regained.

Focal Seizures

Simple partial seizures of motor type (focal motor seizures) may involve the whole limb or part of the limb but do not cause loss of consciousness if the abnormal electrical activity remains localized. Occasionally, movement can march from distal to proximal portions of the limb, such as appearing to move up the arm (over seconds or minutes) into the neck, head, and face. The inability to suppress this movement voluntarily, the duration of more than tens of seconds, and its involvement of abdominal, chest, or neck muscles suggest the epileptic nature.

Simple partial seizures may result in a "rising," poorly describable epigastric discomfort, a sense of internal "shuddering," nausea, malaise, smell, fear, familiarity, or derealization. There may be distortions of vision, with objects appearing smaller, larger, closer, or farther away; distortions of hearing, smell, and feeling; sweating, pupillary dilation, or piloerection. These latter autonomic components are usually seen with other features of partial seizures.

Absence and Complex Partial Seizures

An event characterized by staring and eye blinking, almost as if the patient has interrupted ongoing activity (but without a fall or even dropping of an object held in the hand) is characteristic of an absence (but not a complex partial) seizure. These seizures occur almost exclusively in childhood.

In this case, an electroencephalogram (EEG) (not cerebral imaging) is diagnostic.

If, however, a staring state is accompanied by a look of confusion, fidgeting, wandering, lip smacking, or loss of station, the event is suggestive of a complex partial seizure. These events are characterized by a postictal period of confusion (which may be brief) and are often fewer in number and longer in duration, lasting at least about 30 seconds. The standard of care now usually includes cerebral imaging with a magnetic resonance imaging (MRI) scan for patients with complex partial seizures.

Myoclonic Seizures

Myoclonic seizures outside infancy and early childhood are most frequently seen as part of juvenile myoclonic epilepsy. In this syndrome, usually with onset in adolescence, sudden jerking movements of the hand(s) resulting in dropping of objects, spillages, or breakages are often overlooked or ascribed to clumsiness. Sometimes the history of these events is obtained only as an afterthought after other seizure types have been identified. In juvenile myoclonic epilepsy, the seizure that brings the patient to the physician's attention is usually a tonic-clonic seizure occurring during sleep or shortly after awakening. About one-third of patients may have several seizure types, including absence seizures (staring), myoclonic jerks, and tonic-clonic seizures. An EEG (not cerebral imaging) may be diagnostic.

Other Neurologic Causes of Dizzy Spells

Lightheadedness is a feature often seen with hypoglycemia, posterior circulation TIAs, or psychological dysfunction, and the "company that it keeps" will lead to a correct diagnosis. When seen with vertigo, lightheadedness can represent migraine, drug effects, middle ear dysfunction, or posterior circulation TIAs. Lightheadedness and vertigo are features of so many conditions that, in isolation, they rarely indicate a particular diagnosis. Other neurologic causes of dizzy spells can result from transient disturbances of circulation—either globally, from transient drops of systemic blood pressure, as occurs in syncope and presyncope, or focally, as occurs in a TIA—migraine, metabolic disturbance, or sleep-related disorders.

Transient Ischemic Attacks

With the older population, the physician should keep in mind the possibility of a cerebrovascular cause for dizzy spells. When lightheadedness and malaise are associated with focal weakness, numbness (of one-half of the body, around the mouth), double vision, or distortions in articulated speech, then TIAs should be suspected. The vascular supply to the inner ear can be compromised in a TIA, with vertigo similar to that occurring from disease of the ear. Usually, however, vertigo is not isolated but is accompanied by other features, such as paralysis or numbness of part of the body, or other concerns that would raise the index of suspicion, such as the presence of atrial fibrillation.

If there is transient interruption of blood supply to the reticular activating system in the brainstem, there will be loss of consciousness. This may result from systemic drop of blood pressure, as in Stokes-Adams attacks caused by transient heart block, or from temporary occlusion of the midline basilar artery that supplies the brainstem. Occlusion of other cerebral vessels gives rise to focal neurologic deficits, without loss of consciousness. Tonic-clonic movements are not a usual feature of TIAs but occasionally are seen after emboli to the cerebral cortex.

Vestibular Dizziness

Vertiginous dizziness without lightheadedness brought on by movements of the head suggests a problem of the vestibular apparatus of the ear. A key consideration is that the patient can experience the symptom even while remaining horizontal, unlike those symptomatic from hypotension. Diagnosis of ear pathology is suggested when vertigo is associated with ringing in or recent infection of the ear.

Orthostatic Lightheadedness

If the malaise and lightheadedness occur only within 10 minutes of the patient's rising to the full standing position, then presyncope/syncope from orthostatic hypotension is a probable diagnosis. There is no clear-cut vertigo, but there is often pallor, sweatiness, and a "look of alarm." The patient may reach out in an effort to stabilize an upright position. Similar symptoms, even when the patient is supine, occurring in association with palpitations suggest cardiogenic hypotension from *arrhythmia.* However, palpitation is not always a prominent symptom.

Migraine

Although headache can be seen before, during, and after seizures, spells associated with headache will often be migrainous or psychogenic. In contrast to patients with seizures or TIAs, few *migraine* patients will have impairment of speech, memory, or consciousness, and confusion is rare. Migraine is more gradually progressive than seizures, and consciousness is almost invariably preserved. In *migraine,* there is usually a previous, clearly delineated history of headache with symptoms such as positive visual phenomena (including flashing lights, spots, fortification spectra), nausea, vomiting, phonophobia, and photophobia. In classic cases, abnormalities of either visual or somatic sensation will progress in a characteristic march from the initial site to the final pattern over the course of minutes. As discussed in Chapter 12, such a classic march is the exception rather than the rule. When episodes of visual distortion, malaise, and even mild headache then occur in the same patient, but without nausea, vomiting, or more marked headache, a migraine variant is likely. Conversely, ascribing such complaints to a migraine variant in the absence of a clear migraine history is problematic.

Metabolic Causes

A combination of malaise, sweating, nausea, weakness, and tremulousness is often seen with hypoglycemia. This is most frequently seen in patients on oral hypoglycemic agents or insulin but may also be seen in alcoholism, after gastrointestinal surgery, with liver disease, or after exercise without meals. Hypoglycemic events occasionally trigger tonic-clonic seizures.

A common cause of impaired consciousness with subjective perception of malaise or discomfort and behavioral abnormalities is intoxication with recreational drugs, prescription drugs, or alcohol. It is critical to inquire about the timing of spells in relation to medication or drug intake. If necessary, urine or blood screening for drugs and toxins (tox-screen) can be obtained.

Sleep Disorders

Unexpected body movements suggestive of nocturnal seizures can be associated with normal and abnormal sleep. Narcolepsy is a rare sleep disorder characterized by excessive somnolence and frequent falling asleep. Cataplexy is a sudden loss of body tone with falls brought on by sudden emotion, typically laughter or fright. Narcolepsy may also be accompanied by hallucinations just before sleep or on awakening and a momentary inability to move on awakening (sleep paralysis). During cataplexy (unlike seizures or syncope), the patient remains conscious throughout the fall. The only constant feature of narcolepsy is sleepiness, and the other clinical features may be absent. Sleep-monitoring studies will confirm the diagnosis.

Periodic limb movements of sleep are a nonepileptic cause of arm or leg kicks in adults. These often arouse the patient (or the sleeping partner) from sleep and, because of the repeated interruptions, result in wake-time sleepiness. The leg kicks are slower then those of epilepsy, varying in duration and intensity, and do not occur in wakefulness. Diagnosis can be confirmed with overnight sleep studies.

Frightening dreams and sleep walking may result in alarming nocturnal spells of which the patient is not aware. Episodes can last up to about 30 minutes and usually occur in the first few hours of sleep. There is often coordinated, elaborate, and sustained semipurposeful behavior but not the briefer, typical automatisms of complex partial seizures, such as lip smacking, grunting, picking at clothes, or rapidly repetitive behavior. Children with night terrors may be suddenly aroused from sleep, wild-eyed and screaming usually from stage 3 or 4 sleep. This diagnosis is usually obtained by history alone.

Dizzy Spells Associated with Psychiatric Disturbances

A major challenge to the clinician is determining whether a dizzy spell is psychogenic or neurologic. When the purported trigger or circumstances are highly variable, are bizarre, or wax and wane during the course of the event, the physician should consider a psychogenic cause. A significant number of dizzy spells can have a psychogenic component, and differentiating purely psychogenic, partially psychogenic, and nonpsychogenic events requires skill and patience. However, like medical and neurologic diagnoses, psychiatric diagnoses can be established only by independent criteria. Inability to fit the patient's complaint to a recognized pattern of neurologic or medical disease does not constitute grounds for diagnosing psychogenic dizzy spells. However, certain characteristic patterns suggest that psychiatric inquiry may prove fruitful.

Pseudoseizures

Psychogenic pseudoseizures are nonepileptic events that look like epileptic seizures. Triggered unconsciously by patients who seek attention, pseudoseizures are not malingering, in which the patient makes a deliberate effort to simulate illness to avoid undesired situations, obligations, or work or to obtain disability status. Some of the characteristics of pseudoseizures that help distinguish them from particular seizure types are their longer duration than syncope or epileptic seizures, their variable phenomenology, and their frequent association with emotional situations. Breathing is often deep and purposeful during the spell and may be accompanied by emotional reactions such as laughing or crying and by meaningful speech. If the physician observes an event, he or she should watch for preservation of consciousness, modification of the event in response to external factors (to avoid injury), thrashing (rather than convulsive jerks), pelvic thrusting, or waxing and waning, prolonged limb or body movements. True tonic-clonic seizures are not affected by verbal instruction, but commands may arrest factitious ones.

Some of the most difficult spells to diagnose correctly are psychogenic.

Any constellation of disturbance of apparent sensation, movement, or behavior has been described or seen. Other diagnostic clues to psychogenic spells are "nonanatomic" involvement, such as alternating weakness and jerking; flexion and extension of the limbs; and side-to-side swaying (as opposed to jerking) of the head. Tightly closed eyes that resist opening and biting of the tip (as opposed to the side) of the tongue or of the cheek are suggestive. Most true generalized tonic-clonic seizures last less than two minutes and go through a standard progression without waxing or waning.

Psychogenic events constitute some of the "great imitators" in clinical medicine. Volitional aspects to the event, modification of the event due to external circumstances, or the ability to talk during an apparently generalized seizure suggests a psychogenic cause. More difficult to determine is the psychogenic nature of purely subjective sensations of numbness, malaise, or dizziness. In the absence of other associated features, however, and with a normal examination, reassurance in the first instance is helpful. Many patients with somatization are looking to be reassured that they do not have cancer, brain tumor, or some other deadly disease. Other patients are clearly less easily reassured.

Hyperventilation

Hyperventilation often affects patients with depression or anxiety. Deep respiratory efforts lower the PCO_2, resulting in numbness around the mouth, tingling of the hands, lightheadedness, and confusion. There may be further malaise, anxiety, pallor, and, rarely, unconsciousness. Reassurance sometimes resolves these attacks. The tingling associated with hyperventilation is also discussed in Chapter 10.

Panic Attacks

Panic attacks are characterized by an acute, intense feeling of fear or anxiety and are often accompanied by palpitations, sweating, and a global numbness. Panic attacks often occur with hyperventilation and the attendant clinical features. Their longer duration, preservation of consciousness, and lack of automatisms help distinguish these events from seizures.

Dissociative or Fugue States

Dissociative or fugue states are those in which a patient may wander aimlessly for hours to days. Most patients have had previous psychiatric symptoms. During the attack, the patient appears awake and has a normal waking EEG.

An Approach to the Patient with Dizzy Spells

History

Except for those rare instances in which the examiner is able to witness the dizzy spell, diagnosis is based on the history. The initial differential can sometimes be supported by subsequent findings on physical examination or ancillary testing, but all too often these prove unrevealing.

A careful history of the dizzy spell must include its context, duration, pattern, responsiveness to external stimuli, and regression. The physician should question the patient and witnesses on each point. It is important to use tact in establishing the characteristics of a patient's spell. It is certainly frustrating for the patient and family to have to describe in detail a difficult or alarming experience of which the patient may be only dimly aware. The patient may perceive the physician's tone and course of inquiry as lack of sympathy or understanding and may become defensive, with a subsequent loss of the open communication essential for diagnosis that is based almost exclusively on history.

The physician should always be wary of prepackaged diagnoses. A patient or family may describe events as "petit mal" or "grand mal" or "syncopal" without the event being any of the above. This may be because of a previous medical opinion; because of what family, friends, or witnesses have described; or even to steer (erroneously) the physician in a particular direction. The clinician must base the diagnosis on the available clinical information, not on a previous diagnostic label, which may be outdated or wrong.

The specific details of the history of the event are much more important than the name that patients or witnesses ascribe to the dizzy spell. Of greatest value is the detailed description of particulars of the spell. The inquiry must include a full description of the course of the episode. Particular features of importance are the circumstances immediately before the spell, including the position of the patient or any change in position, and other precipitating factors. These may be identified by the patient and include taking a particular medication or witnessing or undergoing a stressful event (having blood taken, going to the dentist). The physician should inquire after possible precipitants not identified by the patient, such as a relationship to meals, whether the event arises out of sleep, and so forth.

The history should include any observed behavior, its pattern, duration, course, and resolution. The best-quality history includes spontaneous descriptions offered by the patient or witnesses. "You know, it's like when you suddenly get up from a chair and you feel woozy like you're about to faint," or "I felt lightheaded and my vision grayed out, but I didn't fall; then I reached to the wall to support myself." Such descriptions are so classic for presyncope that even a convincing account of subsequent behavior, such as loss of consciousness, a fall, or tonic and clonic movements, even with tongue biting or incontinence, would still steer the examiner toward convulsive syncope rather than a convulsion or tonic-clonic seizure.

The clinician should try to learn from witnesses whether consciousness was preserved and whether there was stiffness or rigidity (an increase in body tone) or floppiness (decrease in body tone). Particular movements or positions of the head, limbs, or body, incontinence, or biting of the tongue is important. Violent muscle contractions occur in tonic-clonic seizures, whereas patients experiencing syncope fall limp.

Of great importance, also, is the rate at which the patient returns to full consciousness. How soon did the patient answer to his or her name or form articulated words with meaning? To better understand this time course, the physician could simulate the chronology of the event by saying "Let's assume the event starts now, and I want you to tell me when [the patient] came around." The examiner can then look at the seconds elapsed on the watch to get a rough estimate as to whether the event lasted seconds or minutes. Often, what was described as five minutes is less than one. Several minutes of confusion are typical after generalized seizures, whereas clarity is quickly regained after syncope.

Usually, the overall pattern of the dizzy spell, rather than any one particular symptom, allows diagnosis. Certain symptoms are common to several types of spells. For example, malaise with lightheadedness may precede syncope or an inner ear problem. To get further into the nature of the event, the examiner should then ask whether the episode included changes in vision (graying out of vision or diplopia), changes in hearing (ringing, deafness), or observable changes in behavior before the fall (staring, fidgeting, eye blinking, lip smacking).

When no witnesses are present for an event that has taken place in the bedroom, inferential information may be obtained by asking about the position of the pillow or bed clothes (bunched up, on the floor, or relatively unchanged), the position of the patient (on the bed, on the floor), whether there was blood on the pillow, whether objects around the bed had been disturbed or knocked off their position, or whether the patient had noticed aching of the limbs in the morning ("as if you had run a mile or had strenuous activity"). Such reports suggest the violent muscular contractions typical of generalized tonic-clonic seizures.

An account from witnesses is of great importance, and sometimes this account is the only one available; on other occasions, the account may differ from that offered by the patient. For example, a lapse in attention may go unnoticed by the patient but not by a family member. An observer may note that the patient stopping activity suddenly to stare, smack or lick his or her lips, pick at clothing, and look confused or dazed.

Physical Examination

The physical examination is most useful when it is directed at finding evidence supporting a diagnosis suggested by the history. If patients describe focal numbness or weakness and speech problems but a preservation of consciousness suggesting TIAs, then the examination should be directed to evidence of cerebrovascular disease. In addition to auscultation of the neck for carotid bruits, the clinician should examine blood pressure in both arms, looking for asymmetry. Pedal pulses should be palpated and the abdominal aorta auscultated, looking for other evidence of atherosclerosis. Auscultation of the heart and determination of the rhythm may reveal sources of cardiogenic emboli. Ophthalmoscopy for emboli or diabetic or hypertensive retinopathy is important, as is auscultation of the closed eye for ocular bruit. A neurologic examination may detect mild persistent deficits either directly related to the described TIA or as evidence of previously completed strokes.

If the symptoms suggest orthostatic hypotension, the clinician should examine the patient's blood pressure and pulse with the patient supine and again after five and ten minutes of standing, taking careful note of any symptoms the patient experiences during this maneuver. If the symptoms suggest vestibular disease, the ears should be examined. Particularly useful are observations of nystagmus, either spontaneously or after the patient has been moved abruptly into a position with the head hanging over the edge of the examining table.

If the patient mentions a bitten tongue, the physician should examine it. If the patient had a fall, the head and body should be examined for evidence of scrapes, bruises, or swelling. When seizures are suspected, a general and neurologic examination may reveal a predisposing disease.

With most dizzy spells, however, the physical and neurologic examinations are often unrevealing. This is not surprising, given the "reversible" nature of a spell. The examination often serves to reassure the patient and physician that other disorders are not present. It is often reassuring to the patient that a "laying on of hands" has been made and that "things have been looked at and examined."

Ancillary Testing

Isolated, brief, and mild dizzy spells rarely need extensive evaluation. They usually do not represent serious disease and resolve spontaneously. Investigation is particularly needed for events that lead to more serious injury, such as broken bones, or for those associated with palpitations or chest pain or a history that suggests TIA or seizure. In deciding on investigation, the physician should consider the following factors: (1) whether a particular diagnosis is serious enough to warrant confirmation or exclusion, (2) the likelihood that a particular test will rule in or exclude a diagnosis, and (3) the risk versus benefit of confirming a particular diagnosis or of the procedure itself. Many investigations, such as angiography, are not without risk to the patient.

It is clear that the "panel" approach to the workup of a particular disorder errs not only by its nonspecificity, but also often by the false belief in its sensitivity: patients with partial epilepsy have a less than 50 percent chance of epileptiform activity on a routine EEG. With increasing health care costs and the push to managed care, a more judicious selection of investigations is being emphasized. Routine blood tests, head computed axial tomograms (CTs), or MRI scans are often unhelpful in identifying the specific cause of "malaise" or loss of consciousness but are routinely done in the emergency setting. Highly sophisticated methods of evaluating causes of spells such as epilepsy monitoring are costly and, when ordered indiscriminately, of low yield. The timing of a test's performance is also of importance. CT head scans (of low yield in patients with transient, mild symptoms) will reveal structural abnormalities that, if present, usually persist over time.

The Role of Electroencephalography

An EEG reflects brain activity only during the time that the EEG is run. Thus, encephalopathy, seizures, and the organic causes of psychiatric diseases are best investigated when the patient is symptomatic. A patient should have an EEG as close as possible to the time of the paroxysmal event, rather than having the test set up several days later as "an outpatient procedure."

Seizures and a diagnosis of epilepsy are usually reached by assessing the patient's history. Short of capturing an actual event on an EEG, there is no absolute diagnostic test. Absence seizures in children may be brought on by hyperventilation or photic stimulation either in the outpatient clinic or, preferably, while an EEG is being run. Many patients with idiopathic generalized epilepsy (previously known as primary generalized epilepsy) may have generalized spike-wave discharges on a routine (interictal) EEG whether they have absence, myoclonic, or tonic-clonic seizures. Patients with focal seizures are less likely to have epileptiform discharges on a routine EEG, and the discharges appear focally. Repeated EEGs, preferably with sleep, have been shown to have an increasing diagnostic yield that plateaus after about five or six EEGs. This should be attempted when the diagnosis remains uncertain (particularly if psychogenic events are considered) and when the patient does not seem to respond to antiepileptic drugs.

It is important to remember that the appearance of isolated epileptic discharges on EEG does not confirm that a particular event is epileptic in nature, since patients with epilepsy may have dizzy spells due to other causes. Nonetheless, epileptiform discharges have a high correlation with epilepsies.

When the Diagnosis Is Uncertain

When the physician suspects seizures or epilepsy but the patient does not respond to antiepileptic drugs and repeated outpatient EEGs are negative, the condition may be psychogenic. Inpatient video-EEG recording or outpatient ambulatory EEG may capture a dizzy spell. If the video shows a "typical" spell according to the patient's family or witnesses and is not accompanied by EEG changes, the event is usually psychogenic. Ambulatory EEG is somewhat less available and is often more affected by artifact from the patient's movement or disconnected electrodes that will not be seen without a video correlate. Home videos by the patient's parents or family members can often be of great help in distinguishing behavioral from organic spells.

The physician should resist applying a label like "epilepsy" or "epileptic seizures" to patients whose diagnosis is in doubt. When labeled as such, patients may lose driving privileges, lose their job, and suffer financial and social problems. Rather then risking an incorrect diagnosis of epilepsy, the physician might best await more information. In the interim, reassuring the patient, explaining the diagnostic process, and awaiting further dizzy spells can be the best course.

Summary

The key to the diagnosis and subsequent management of dizzy spells is an accurate history. Specific knowledge of the precise details of the incident, of the patient's subjective experience, and of the observations of witnesses is required. These details will allow the assignment of most spells to specific categories, the most important of which are seizures, transient ischemic attacks, vestibular disturbances, and hypotension. Spells whose description does not fit one of these major categories should prompt consideration of more unusual causes: sleep disorders, fugue states, migraine, pseudoseizures, and metabolic disturbance. Physical examination can reproduce symptoms and signs of vestibular disturbance and orthostatic hypotension but either is nonrevealing or serves as an indirect pointer to associated disease in most other cases. Laboratory evaluation can in some instances provide confirmatory support but is rarely revealing in the absence of a clear clinical hypothesis. In many instances, management depends on a clinical diagnosis established by consideration of history alone.

REFERENCES

Commission on Classification and Terminology of the International League against Epilepsy. Proposal for Revised Clinical and Electroencephalographic Classification of Epileptic Seizures. *Epilepsia* 22 (1981): 489.

Harper, M., and Roth, M. Temporal Lobe Epilepsy and the Phobic Anxiety-Depersonalization Syndrome: Part 1. A Comparative Study. *Comprehensive Psychiatry* 3 (1962): 129–151.

Strub, R. L. Dizziness. In *Decision Making in Adult Neurology,* edited by L. A. Weisberg, R. L. Strub, and C. A. Garcia, pp. 54–55. Philadelphia: B. C. Decker, 1987.

Weisberg, L. A. Transient Ischemic Attack: Carotid. In *Decision Making in Adult Neurology,* edited by L. A. Weisberg, R. L. Strub, and C. A. Garcia, pp. 102–103. Philadelphia: B. C. Decker, 1987.

————. Transient Ischemic Attack: Vertebrobasilar. In *Decision Making in Adult Neurology,* edited by L. A. Weisberg, R. L. Strub, and C. A. Garcia, pp. 104–105. Philadelphia: B. C. Decker, 1987.

FOURTEEN

Tremor

Stephen G. Reich, M.D.

Tremor is commonly encountered in primary care. For some patients it interferes with activities of daily living. Others are concerned about a serious underlying disease, such as Parkinson disease. For some, tremor is a source of embarrassment or an incidental finding. With simple techniques of history and physical examination, the primary care physician can make the correct diagnosis and determine when to initiate treatment, pursue further workup, or refer to a specialist.

The Classification of Tremor

A *tremor* is a rhythmic oscillation of a body part. The rhythmic nature of tremor distinguishes it from other involuntary movement disorders, such as chorea, dystonia, myoclonus, or motor tics, which are not rhythmic. Tremor can either be physiologic or pathologic. The differential diagnosis almost always boils down to essential tremor (ET) or Parkinson disease (PD) after a few notable exceptions such as drug-induced tremor, hyperthyroidism, and Wilson disease have been ruled out. There are other much less common types, such as cerebellar tremor, primary writing tremor, and orthostatic tremor.

The three most helpful characteristics that distinguish different types of tremor are the position of maximum activation, frequency, and associated neurologic signs. A tremor most activated at *rest* and reduced with movement or maintenance of posture is characteristic of PD. Conversely, essential tremor and enhanced physiologic tremor are maximally activated with maintenance of a *posture* (arms held in front or bent at the elbows in front of the nose) and commonly persist throughout movement. *Kinetic* tremor (or what used to be called intention tremor) is activated with *purposeful movement* and is characteristic of cerebellar disease. Although cerebellar and essential tremor are both activated with movement, only cerebellar tremor increases in amplitude as the target is approached.

Frequency also aids classification of tremor but less reliably. It is difficult to estimate frequency accurately at the bedside. The cerebellar tremor is slowest, generally 3–5 Hz (cycles per second), overlapping with the slow to medium frequency of the parkinsonian rest tremor, 3–6 Hz. ET is medium to fast in frequency, 6–12 Hz, with the fastest frequencies suggesting enhanced physiologic tremor. Associated signs include bradykinesia and rigidity in PD and incoordination in cerebellar disease, whereas essential tremor is a monosymptomatic disorder—lacking in associated signs.

Specific Types of Tremor

Everyone has a slight tremor of the outstretched hands that is usually not apparent. But under certain circumstances, this physiologic tremor may become symptomatic, or *enhanced* (Table 14.1). Such enhancement is normal after carrying a heavy bag of groceries or when nervous, hungry, cold, or febrile. These short-lived, situational tremors rarely come to medical attention. A similar tremor is often seen in the setting of drug and alcohol withdrawal or accompanying acute metabolic derangements such as hypoglycemia or hyponatremia, and it disappears when the offending insult is resolved.

Table 14.1. Drugs and Other Factors That Enhance Physiologic Tremor

Drugs	Alcohol and drug withdrawal
Lithium	Anxiety
Antipsychotics	Postexercise/exertion
Valproic acid	Metabolic derangements
Corticosteroids	Hyperthyroidism
Tricyclic antidepressants	Hypoglycemia
Beta-adrenergic agonists	Hyponatremia
Theophylline	Pheochromocytoma
Others	Hypothermia

A more persistent enhanced physiologic tremor can be seen with many prescription medications or with hyperthyroidism and, unlike the above, may bring the patient to medical attention. More often than not, it proves to be an asymptomatic physical finding. If patients on theophylline, lithium, valproic acid, or tricyclic antidepressants (among others) extend their arms, most will have a subtle tremor of very low amplitude (less than 1 cm) and high frequency.

In all patients with a postural or kinetic tremor, (1) take a drug history, (2) check thyroid function, and (3) consider screening for Wilson disease, unless another cause is readily apparent. The diagnosis of an enhanced physiologic tremor is confirmed if the tremor disappears after the offending drug, situation, or metabolic abnormality is withdrawn or corrected. If the tremor persists, then it is reasonable to conclude that the patient has ET, which can also be exacerbated by the same precipitants. When medication cannot be withdrawn, as in the well-controlled manic-depressive patient on lithium, a symptomatic enhanced physiologic tremor can be treated like ET, as will be discussed below.

Distinguishing Essential Tremor from Parkinson Disease

The prognosis and treatment of tremor depend on careful diagnosis. ET is a *monosymptomatic* disorder that progresses insidiously over years to decades, if at all. In contrast, PD is a progressive neurodegenerative disorder. Although tremor is the most common presenting symptom of PD, up to one-third of people with PD have no tremor. Distinguishing ET from PD can be accomplished by considering a few clinical characteristics (Table 14.2). During history taking, the physician should determine the patient's age at onset, duration of symptoms, part(s) of the body affected by tremor, medications taken, family history, and response of the tremor to alcohol. In preparation for deciding on therapy and assessing its results, the physician needs to know the effect of tremor on the activities of daily living and whether it is a source of psychological distress, primarily embarrassment.

In the physical examination, determine what parts of the body are

Table 14.2. Parkinson Disease versus Essential Tremor

	Parkinson Disease	Essential Tremor
History		
Age of onset (yr)	60, with limited variability	Variable, more common after 50
Duration of symptoms before presentation	Months to 1 yr	Years to decades
Family history	Generally negative	Generally positive (autosomal dominant)
Response to alcohol (small amount)	Little or none	Improvement
Physical examination		
Position of maximal activation	Rest	Maintenance of a posture and movement
Frequency	3–6 Hz	6–12 Hz
Morphology	Pill-rolling	Flexion-extension at shoulder, wrist
Onset	Unilateral	Bilateral, may be asymmetric
Body part affected	Upper limb > lower limb > chin = lips	Upper limbs > head > voice > chin = lips > lower limbs
Handwriting	Small, no tremor	Normal size, tremulous
Natural history	Progressive	Insidiously progressive, may seem to plateau

affected by the tremor (hands, legs, head, voice, other), the position of max-imal activation, tremor frequency (slow, medium, or fast), the look or mor-phology of the tremor, and associated signs (e.g., bradykinesia, incoordi-nation, etc.). Last, obtain a sample of the patient's handwriting and have the patient draw a spiral.

Consider two illustrative cases: which one has ET and which one has PD?

Case Example: A 48-year-old man presents for evaluation of tremor of both hands. He recalls intermittent shaking as long as twenty years ago, which over the years progressed insidiously to the point where he is now having diffi-culty performing dexterous tasks, particularly writing. His mother and ma-ternal uncle both have tremor. He has noticed that the tremor "settles down" after a glass of wine. On examination, the upper limbs are quiet at rest. There is a tremor of both upper extremities when outstretched, and it persists with finger-to-nose movement. A handwriting sample shows tremulous writing, and tremor also shows when the patient draws a spiral (Fig. 14.1). The rest of the examination is normal.

Case Example: A 58-year-old woman presents for evaluation of tremor of the right (dominant) hand. It began a little less than a year ago. Others have com-mented that she doesn't swing her right arm while walking, and she has no-a

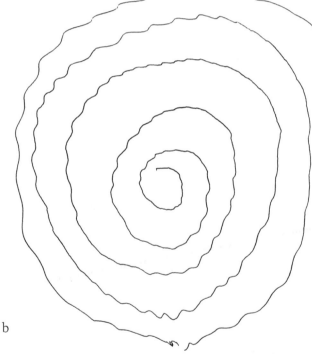

b

Figure 14.1. (a) Samples of handwriting demonstrate micrographia but no tremor (patient with Parkinson disease—*top*) and normal size but tremulous writing (patient with essential tremor—*bottom*). Each patient has written "Today is a nice day in Baltimore." (b) Typical pattern of rhythmic oscillations of the pen, characteristic of essential tremor.

ticed a tendency to drag the right leg. Her handwriting has become smaller. She has observed that all movements with the right hand are slower and that she has difficulty arising from a low chair and turning in bed. On examination, there is diminished blink rate and facial expression. Her voice is a bit soft. There is a slow tremor at rest of the right hand. Rapid repetitive movements of the right hand and foot are slow and crowded together. There is mild cogwheel rigidity in the right arm and slight cogwheel rigidity in the left. She walks a bit slow, with absent arm swing on the right.

History

Age of onset can provide a helpful clue to distinguish between PD and ET, although there is considerable overlap. Most people with PD present between age 55 and 65. ET, while increasing in incidence with age, may begin in childhood and not uncommonly presents in the third, fourth, or fifth decade, which would be unusual for PD. At the far end of the age spectrum, ET is again much more common, hence the designation *senile tremor,* a term that has largely been abandoned. More helpful than age of onset is *duration.* In general, most people with PD present within a year of the onset of tremor, whereas those with ET often present several years or even decades after onset.

PD almost always begins as *hemi*-PD with a unilateral tremor of the upper limb, unrelated to handedness. In contrast, ET is almost always bilateral at onset but may be asymmetrical, typically of greater amplitude in the dominant hand. A tremor of the head or voice is almost always ET. Whereas both types of tremor may involve the lips, chin, or tongue, these areas are more commonly affected in Parkinson disease. It is not uncommon for a person to notice only tremor of the hand(s) and be unaware of involvement of other body parts, which is apparent during examination.

Alcohol often reduces ET, whereas it typically has little or no effect on the tremor of PD. Only a small amount of alcohol is necessary to suppress ET temporarily, and many patients find this a helpful "treatment" when used judiciously. There does not seem to be an increased incidence of alcoholism in people with ET.

A strong family history points in the direction of ET, but ET can also be sporadic. Many patients with ET will initially deny having an affected relative. That their mother or father was "trembly" toward the end of life may have been passed off and forgotten as simply "old age." The physician should ask whether anyone in the family has or had tremulous handwriting, a quiver of the voice, or tremor of the head. Sometimes patients will report a parent or other first-degree relative had "Parkinson disease" when, indeed, the person had ET, especially if the "Parkinson disease" included tremor of the head or voice or was unaccompanied by slowness of movement or difficulty walking.

Finally, ask how the patient is affected, both physically and psychologically, by the tremor. Although this information may help to distinguish ET from PD, it is most useful for deciding whether treatment is necessary and for assessing its effectiveness. Since the rest tremor of PD typically suppresses with movement, most patients do not find that it interferes significantly with their functioning, whereas slowness and incoordination do. In contrast, by the time most people with ET seek medical attention, tremor has started to interfere with many routine dexterous tasks. Equally troublesome are psychological effects, primarily embarrassment. Many people with tremor avoid social interactions, and those with ET of the voice often shy away from public speaking or talking on the telephone. It is important for the physician specifically to ask patients whether they are embarrassed, since, paradoxically, they are often too embarrassed to admit it! After taking a directed history, the physician can almost always recognize whether the patient has ET or PD. Go back and look at the two cases above. Who has ET and who has PD?

Physical Examination

The distinction between ET and PD is confirmed by physical examination. Usually both types of tremor involve the upper extremities. Begin by looking to see whether the tremor is maximally activated with the patient's hands resting comfortably on his or her lap, with arms extended, or with purposeful movements—finger to nose or drinking from a cup. In PD, the tremor is most obvious at rest. Next, observe whether the tremor frequency is slow, as in PD, or medium fast, as in ET. Finally, observe the *look* or morphology of the tremor. With PD, this is typically ab- and adduction of the thumb, with flexion-extension of the fingers, as though rolling a pill, hence the name "pill-rolling." Sometimes, the morphology is more of a grasping movement between the thumb and fingers or pronation-supination of the forearm. ET is primarily a flexion-extension movement at the shoulder, wrist, or fingers.

An exclusively unilateral tremor is almost always going to be PD. With time, though (often several years), the tremor does spread to the opposite side of the body. In contrast, ET is almost always bilateral at onset (though occasionally asymmetric, with greater amplitude in the dominant hand). Although both most commonly affect the upper limbs, the involvement of other body parts is another helpful clue. ET is uncommon in the lower extremities, whereas PD may begin in one foot. Tremor of the head or voice is almost always ET and not PD. Tremor of the lips, tongue, or chin can be seen with either but is more common with PD.

Having a patient write a sentence and draw a spiral is the next step. The tremor of PD is usually suppressed with voluntary activity but the handwriting is small when the dominant hand is involved. In early disease, micrographia may occur only at the end of a long word: BALTIMORE. Reviewing the patient's checkbook entries is another helpful way of documenting progressively smaller writing. In ET, the size of the handwriting is unaffected, but tremor is evident in handwriting and also when drawing a spiral.

The physician concludes the examination by looking for associated neurologic signs. In ET, tremor is usually the only abnormality. The exception, which sometimes causes confusion, is that cogwheel rigidity, while a cardinal feature of PD, may also be seen with ET and, by itself, cannot differentiate the two. Early PD is characterized by other signs not seen with ET, including bradykinesia (slowness of movement), decreased arm swing, diminished facial expression and blink rate, a monotone and soft voice, shuffling gait, flexed posture, and hesitation when arising from a chair, among others (Table 14.3).

If, after completing the history taking and physical examination outlined above, the diagnosis is still not clear, the primary care physician should refer the patient to a neurologist for confirmation.

Table 14.3. Symptoms and Signs in Parkinson Disease

Cardinal Signs	Psychological Symptoms
Bradykinesia	Bradyphrenia
Rest tremor	Anxiety
Cogwheel rigidity	Dementia
Additional Motor Signs	Depression
Micrographia	Autonomic Symptoms and Signs
Difficulty turning in bed	Orthostatic hypotension
Decreased arm swing	Constipation
Difficulty arising from a deep	Urinary bladder instability
chair/car/toilet, etc.	Impotence/impaired arousal response in
Impaired dexterity	women
Hypomimia	Altered thermoregulation
Hypophonia	Sweating
Chin/tongue tremor	Dysphagia
Flexed posture	Drooling
En bloc turning	Other
Start hesitation/freezing	Seborrhea
Festination	Sleep disturbance
Retropulsion/impaired postural	Fatigue
righting reflexes	
Sensory Symptoms	
Pain	
Paresthesia	
Restless legs syndrome	
Akathisia	

The Management of Essential Tremor

The first step in the treatment of ET is education and reassurance. Many patients with ET are worried that they have PD or another serious disorder. They should also be informed that the tremor is not a sign that they are anxious, even though they have probably already observed exacerbation of the tremor when nervous. The physician should emphasize the insidious progression and that ET is not a degenerative disorder. For most but not all affected persons, ET is no more than a nuisance. It is often useful to bring the frequently used designation *benign* ET into this discussion. Yet, for some patients, ET can significantly interfere with functioning and is far from benign. The physician should refer all patients to the International Tremor Foundation for additional education and support and for research updates (International Tremor Foundation, 7046 West 105th Street, Overland Park, KN 66212-1803; phone 913-341-3880, fax 913-341-1296).

Whether treatment is necessary hinges largely on how much the tremor interferes with the patient's activities of daily living (ADLs). Can the person write? use a computer mouse? button clothing? use eating utensils? eat soup? apply makeup? fasten jewelry? shave? put toothpaste on the toothbrush? When these and similar activities are compromised, treatment is indicated. An occasional patient with little functional impairment will want treatment because of embarrassment, which in some cases can be as limiting as the physical effects of ET. At the outset, the physician should advise the patient that no medication will *cure* the tremor. The goal of treatment is to reduce the tremor and improve functioning. The effectiveness of treatment is judged by assessing the ADLs at each visit.

The two first-line drugs for ET are the anticonvulsant primidone and the beta blocker propranolol. Both are efficacious and most helpful for tremor of the upper limb rather than tremor of the head or voice. Begin treatment with 25 mg of primidone at night (it comes in 50- and 250-mg scored tablets). About 5 percent of patients will experience the well-documented but poorly understood *first-dose phenomenon*. The day after this homeopathic dose, they feel terrible: nauseated, dizzy, fatigued, and confused. Although frightening, it is short-lived, self-limited, and not a contraindication to restarting therapy after this effect has worn off. If prepared, most patients can weather this brief but often upsetting storm. Equally uncommon but as dramatic is the occasional patient who reports a marked improvement on this low dose. For most, a higher dose is needed.

Escalate by 25 mg approximately every five days to an initial maintenance dose of 50 mg bid. If needed, continue to escalate slowly to 100 mg tid. If there is no improvement whatsoever on that dose, there is usually little to be gained from higher doses, though one can go as high as 250 mg tid. It is not necessary to check blood levels (primidone or its metabolite, phenobarbital) unless there is concern about clinical toxicity or compliance. The most common side effects include sedation, imbalance, impaired concentration, and occasional depression. These often improve after prolonged use.

If the maximally tolerated dose of primidone affords some but insufficient improvement, then *add* propranolol because the two are synergistic. If there is *no* improvement with primidone, then slowly taper it off and substitute propranolol. During the taper, many patients will notice exacerbation of the tremor, demonstrating that the primidone was more effective than originally appreciated. If so, continue it at the lowest dose that seemed to offer benefit.

Propranolol is as effective as primidone for ET. In young patients, consider beginning with Inderal LA, 60 mg. In elderly patients, a more homeopathic approach is recommended: start with 10 or 20 mg once per day. In each case, the dose is escalated gradually, aiming for satisfactory tremor control (not a cure) without intolerable side effects, to a maximal daily dosage of 320 mg. Contraindications to the use of a beta blocker include reactive airways disease, brittle diabetes, congestive heart failure, and heart block. Other beta blockers, including metoprolol (the preferred choice in the patient with reactive airways disease because of its preferential, relative beta 1 antagonism) and nadolol, have also been shown to be effective for ET, but none is superior to propranolol.

Some patients desire treatment only on an as-needed basis (e.g., before public speaking or a social engagement). Many times they have already learned on their own that a small amount of alcohol is helpful in this setting, and this is an effective treatment as long as it does not lead to abuse, which rarely occurs. Other drugs that can be used include the short-acting benzodiazepine alprazolam or propranolol.

Not infrequently, patients continue to have a bothersome tremor despite maximal doses of primidone and propranolol, even in combination. A second-line drug is clonazepam; begin with 0.25 mg at night and slowly escalate until either adequate control or intolerance. If it, like the first-line drugs, is ineffective, then it is unlikely that other medications will work. At this point, referral to a specialist is indicated.

Specialist Treatment of Essential Tremor

Botulinum toxin is another option for ET and is usually of greater benefit for tremor of the head or voice compared to its limited effectiveness for the upper limb. For ET of the head, botulinum toxin is most effective when the movement is horizontal. For ET of the voice, it can be injected into the vocal cords; although this may cause mild, transient hypophonia or dysphagia, these problems usually resolve within several weeks after the injection. The beneficial effect tends to wane after four months, requiring a repeat injection. Only an experienced practitioner should inject botulinum toxin.

Two surgical procedures are available for the treatment of severe ET of the upper limbs and are equally helpful for parkinsonian tremor: stereotactic thalamotomy and deep-brain stimulation (DBS) of the thalamus. Each procedure has advantages and disadvantages, and a full discussion is beyond the scope of this chapter, except to mention that thalamotomy should be avoided in the patient who requires a bilateral procedure because of the risk of dysarthria. Both procedures are highly effective for either curing or substantially reducing tremor contralateral to the operated side, and the risk of a serious complication is low. Unlike thalamotomy, DBS can be performed safely bilaterally. The physician should refer appropriate candidates to a center experienced in surgical treatment of tremor and, ideally, one where there is close collaboration between the neurosurgeon and a neurologist with expertise in movement disorders.

The Treatment of Parkinson Disease

Many of the principles suggested for the treatment of ET also apply to PD. Since the tremor of PD often attenuates with movement, it tends to cause little functional impairment but can be a source of embarrassment. Generally, the other features of PD, notably bradykinesia, dictate the need for treatment based on the patient's functional status. Furthermore, antiparkinsonian medications often have little effect on tremor. Nevertheless, there is often some, albeit modest, improvement with anticholinergics, levodopa, amantadine, or dopamine agonists. A full discussion of the treatment of PD is not practical here and is given in the references.

A small percentage of people with PD have a disabling tremor that no longer appears exclusively at rest but persists with maintenance of posture and movement, significantly affecting functioning. Sometimes the medications used for ET are helpful in this situation, but when they are not, these patients are candidates for thalamotomy or DBS of the thalamus.

Cerebellar Tremor

Although tremor is a common feature of cerebellar disease, it is rare for such patients to present with tremor as the predominant symptom; their concern is typically incoordination, imbalance, or difficulty walking. If the presenting complaint is tremor, be wary of diagnosing cerebellar disease. Remember also that ET, while classically a postural tremor, on occasion may appear exclusively or predominantly with movement (the *kinetic variant*) and may be mistakenly called a cerebellar tremor.

The tremor of cerebellar disease is slow, somewhat irregular, and maximally activated with movement. It increases in amplitude as the target is approached, hence the term *intention tremor* (now replaced by *kinetic tremor*), and it may also be present with maintenance of a posture. A cerebellar tremor is virtually always accompanied by other cerebellar signs that support the diagnosis. These include incoordination of rapid alternating movements (dysdiadokokinesia); inaccuracy of purposeful movements (dysmetria); irregular variations in the volume and rhythm of speech (scanning speech); a broad-based, reeling gait ("like a drunken sailor"); quasi-rhythmical rocking of the head or trunk (titubation); hypotonia; and nystagmus and other ocular motor abnormalities.

The multitude of diseases and conditions affecting the cerebellum can be broadly divided into acquired and degenerative. Patients with the latter typically present with a gait disorder and incoordination, and tremor is rarely a prominent part of the picture. The most severe cerebellar tremors are encountered in acquired diseases. In these situations, the diagnosis is often obvious: head trauma, multiple sclerosis, or a posterior circulation stroke. Accurate diagnosis, which may require referral to a neurologist, is essential.

Treatment is usually directed at the underlying disease, rather than the tremor itself. Occasionally, applying a weight to the limb will suppress the tremor slightly, but short of surgery, little else has been shown to work for cerebellar tremor. For the patient with a disabling cerebellar tremor, consider surgical therapy. While beneficial, the degree and duration of improvement is often less than that experienced with surgical treatment of ET or PD.

Miscellaneous Tremors

Primary Writing Tremor

Primary writing tremor is part of a larger category of *task-specific* movement disorders that are characterized by the appearance of an involuntary movement only or at least predominantly during a specific task. Patients with primary writing tremor experience shaking of the hand when writing, yet, surprisingly, they are able to carry out other equally dexterous tasks and maintain posture with little or no tremor. Closely related is *dystonic writer's cramp,* a task-specific form of dystonia, which is a syndrome of sustained, stereotyped muscle spasms causing twisting or turning movements or abnormal postures. Some patients with dystonic writer's cramp have an associated tremor, often referred to as a *dystonic tremor.* Many patients adapt by using pencils rather than pens, using wider writing instruments, or holding writing instruments in a unique manner—for instance, gripping a pencil in the palm as though holding an ice pick.

People who have writing tremor often respond to medications used for ET. When tremor is accompanied by a mild degree of dystonia, anticholinergics and other agents used for focal dystonias may be successful. Although botulinum toxin is often helpful for simple, mild forms of dystonic writer's cramp, the results with primary writing tremor are often disappointing. If primary writing tremor becomes so severe as to jeopardize a person's occupation, then consider surgical treatment.

Primary Orthostatic Tremor

People with primary orthostatic tremor relate the unique history that they "can't stand still" even though they are able to sit, walk, and run without difficulty. The initial step in the diagnosis is to be aware of this disorder and recognize the characteristic history. On examination, it is critical to watch what happens when the patient stands: the tremor may take as long as a minute to appear, at which point there is a low-amplitude, slightly irregular, high-frequency tremor of the legs; then patients typically become very anxious and unsteady and insist that they have urgently either to walk or to sit. When the tremor is of very low amplitude, it may be detected more easily with palpation rather than inspection. Some cases are diagnosed only by electromyography. However, it is rarely necessary to go to such lengths to make a diagnosis, since few other conditions need be considered in the differential for a patient who can walk well but cannot stand. Clonazepam is the first-line treatment. However, when it is poorly tolerated or ineffective, medications used for ET may prove useful, as may gabapentin and levodopa.

Wilson Disease

Although ET and PD are far and away the most common tremors encountered, always remember three important *rule-outs:* drug-induced tremor, hyperthyroidism, and Wilson disease. This rare, autosomal recessive disorder is due to a defect in copper transport, leading to toxic accumulation. The most common sites of involvement include the liver and basal ganglia, and tremor, of any type, may be a manifestation of the latter. The classic tremor of Wilson disease is of large amplitude and proximal, often described as "wing beating," but it may cause a rest or kinetic tremor often accompanied by other involuntary movements such as bradykinesia and dystonia. The neurologic presentation also commonly includes dysarthria, drooling, and psychiatric symptoms.

Although Wilson disease is a zebra, it is worth always keeping in mind. When therapy is instituted early, it can halt the progression and reverse many of the symptoms and signs. However, if diagnosis and treatment are delayed, there is inexorable and sometimes irreversible progression. Unfortunately, the diagnosis is often delayed primarily because Wilson disease simply is not considered. It deserves consideration in all patients younger than 50 with a tremor, and indeed *any* movement disorder.

Although it is unrealistic to screen every patient with a movement disorder for Wilson disease, it is prudent at least to have a low threshold for testing. If a tremor fits easily into one of the known categories, such as ET or PD, and has been present for several years with no atypical neurologic or systemic features and a negative family history for Wilson disease, such testing is not appropriate. For almost everyone else, though, particularly those below the age of 30, consider Wilson disease. The screen involves measuring serum ceruloplasmin, which will be low in at least 90 percent of cases; a 24-hour urine collection for copper, which is elevated in Wilson disease; and referral to an ophthalmologist for a slit-lamp examination to search for a Kayser-Fleischer ring. If these tests are positive or if the clinical suspicion of Wilson disease remains high despite equivocal or negative testing, refer the patient to a center with expertise in Wilson disease.

Summary

Most types of tremor can be diagnosed by a focused history and physical examination. The differential diagnosis is almost always between Parkinson disease and essential tremor, which have different prognoses and respond to different medications. These are distinguished by the characteristics of the tremor and the presence or absence of associated signs. Duration since onset and other historical features can also provide helpful clues. Essential tremor must be distinguished from enhanced physiologic tremor resulting from medications or hyperthyroidism. Wilson disease should be considered in all young persons with tremor. The history and physical examination are also sufficient for the diagnosis of cerebellar tremor, as well as rarer entities such as primary writing tremor and primary orthostatic tremor. Treatment is available for most types of tremor, including surgery for those with severe tremor refractory to medications.

REFERENCES

Bain, P. G. The Effectiveness of Treatments for Essential Tremor. *The Neurologist* 5 (1997): 305–321.

Cleeves, L.; Findley, L. J.; and Marsden, C. D. Odd Tremors. In *Movement Disorders 3,* edited by C. D. Marsden and S. Fahn, pp. 434–458. Oxford: Butterworth-Heinemann, 1994.

Deuschl, G.; Bain, P.; and Brin, M. Consensus Statement of the Movement Disorder Society on Tremor. *Movement Disorders* 13 (1998): 2–23.

Elble, R. J., and Koller, W. C. *Tremor.* Baltimore: Johns Hopkins University Press, 1990.

Findley, L. J., and Koller, W. C. Essential Tremor: A Review. *Neurology* 37 (1987): 1194–1197.

Fink, John K.; Hedera, Peter; and Brewer, George J. Hepatolenticular Degeneration (Wilson's Disease). *The Neurologist* 5 (1999): 171–185.

Hallett, Mark. Classification and Treatment of Tremor. *Journal of the American Medical Association* 266 (1991): 1115–1117.

Heilman, K. M. Orthostatic Tremor. *Archives of Neurology* 41 (1984): 880–881.

Koller, W.; Pahwa, R.; Busenbark, K.; Hubble, J.; Wilkinson, S.; Lang, A.; Tuite, P.; Sime, E.; Lazan Malapira, T.; Smith, D.; Tarsy, D.; Miyawaki, E.; Norregaard, T.; Kormos, T.; and Olanow, C. W. High-Frequency Unilateral Thalamic Stimulation in the Treatment of Essential and Parkinsonian Tremor. *Annals of Neurology* 42 (1997): 292–299.

Lang, A. E., and Lozano, A. M. Parkinson's Disease. *New England Journal of Medicine* 339 (1998): 1044–1053, 1130–1143.

Mendis, T.; Suchowersky, O.; Lang, A.; and Gauthier, S. Management of Parkinson's Disease: A Review of Current and New Therapies. *Canadian Journal of Neurological Sciences* 26 (1999): 89–103.

Rosenbaum, F., and Jankovic, J. Focal Task-specific Tremor and Dystonia: Categorization of Occupational Movement Disorders. *Neurology* 38 (1998): 522–527.

Schuurman, P. R.; Bosch, D. A.; Bossuyt, P. M.; Bonsel, G. J.; van Someren, E. J.; de Bie, R. M.; and Merkus, A. Comparison of Continuous Thalamic Stimulation and Thalamotomy for Suppression of Severe Tremor. *New England Journal of Medicine* 342 (2000): 461–468.

Zirh, A.; Lenz, F. A.; Reich, S. G.; Rowland, L. H.; and Dougherty, P. M. Stereotactic Thalamotomy in the Treatment of Essential Tremor: Re-assessment Including a Blinded Measure of Outcome. *Journal of Neurology, Neurosurgery and Psychiatry* 66 (1999): 772–775.

Index

Abstinence syndrome, 96, 113
Acetazolamide, 181
Adjustment disorder with depressed mood, 12-13
Agnosia. See Focal cognitive syndromes
Agoraphobia, 38, 69
AIDS. See Human immunodeficiency virus
Alcohol: abstinence syndrome, 96; abuse, group treatment, 115–16, 118–19; —, laboratory results suggesting, 102, 103; —, and major depression in women, 115, 119; —, in panic disorder, 39; —, physical signs of, 102; —, and small-fiber neuropathy, 133; —, in social phobia, 40; abuse liability of, 94–95; amnestic syndrome due to, 54, 63; craving for, 99, 117–18; cross-tolerance to opioids of, 99, 122; delirium due to, 53; detoxification from, 106–9; disulfiram to prevent use of, 107, 116–17, 121; essential tremor affected by, 219, 224; as headache trigger, 180; insomnia after detoxification from, 116; naltrexone hydrochloride for craving of, 117–18, 121; "predrinking" of, 99; risk factors with, 101; tremor in withdrawal from, 215; suicide and, 80, 85; weakness due to, 145; withdrawal potential of, 95, 100
Alcoholics Anonymous, 115–16, 118–19
Allodynia, 157
Alprazolam: avoiding for panic disorder, 45; detoxification from, 114; for essential tremor, 224; toxicology screen for, 103; withdrawal potential of, 45, 95, 112
Alzheimer Association, 62
Alzheimer disease. See Dementia
Amnesia: causes of, 46, 54; as focal cognitive syndrome, 52; and hippocampal damage, 135; transient global in migraine, 185; treatment of, 63–64
Amphetamine: abuse liability of, 94; as migraine trigger, 189; withdrawal from, 17
Amyotrophic lateral sclerosis, 146–47, 151, 152
Anemia: dementia caused by, 53; mimicking anxiety disorder, 40
Anesthesia: injury from, 157, 165, 168; saddle, 159, 162
Antidepressants: bupropion hydrochloride, 109–10; choosing among, 31–32; for cocaine abuse, 109–10, 120; for generalized anxiety disorder, 43–44, 120; for major depression, 24–33, 90, 109–10; selective

serotonin reuptake inhibitors, 27–29, 31, 32, 43–44, 90; suicide risk increasing, 90; tremor from, 216; tricyclic, 25–27, 31, 32, 45, 52–53, 90, 109, 190–91, 216; venlafaxine hydrochloride, 30–31
Anxiety: normal, 35; subsyndromal, 37
Anxiety disorders: and alcohol abuse in women, 115; course of, 48–49; epidemiology of, 36–37, 39, 69; excluding medical disorders in, 40–41; explaining diagnosis to patients, 42–43; generalized anxiety disorder, 37–38, 43–44, 48; hyperventilation in numbness and tingling, 158; and major depression, 19, 38, 39; obsessive-compulsive disorder, 39–40, 47, 49; panic disorder, 38–39, 40, 45–47, 48–49, 69, 158, 206; referral to specialists for, 47–48; screening for, 41–42; social phobia, 40, 47, 49; somatic symptoms in, 36, 37, 38, 39, 66, 68–69; treatment of, 42–49, 113
Aphasia: causes of, 54; in dementia, 53–54; as focal cognitive syndrome, 52; and hemispheric lesions, 134–35, 135–36; treatment of, 63
Apraxia. See Focal cognitive syndromes
Arrhythmia, cardiac: anxiety disorders mimicked by, 40; dizziness due to, 202, 203
Arteritis, temporal. See Headaches
Ataxia: with cerebellar tremor, 226; examination for, 142; as posterior fossa lesion sign, 134. See also Cerebellum; Coordination; Tremor
Azidothymidine, 145

Back pain: compression fracture causing, 173–74; evaluation of, 172–74; mechanics of, 171–72; prevalence of, 171; specialist referral for, 172–77; treatment of, 115, 174–77. See also Cauda equina syndrome; Disc, herniated
Baclofen, 182
Barbiturates: abstinence syndrome from, 96; abuse liability of, 94; cross-tolerance with benzodiazepines of, 122; delirium due to, 53; detoxification from, 114–15; duration of action of, 114; physical signs of abuse, 102; toxicology screen for, 103; withdrawal potential of, 95. See also Phenobarbital; Primidone; Psychoactive substances
Baresthesia, 166

Basal ganglia, damage to, 135
"BATHE" screening interview, 41–42
Benzodiazepines: abstinence syndrome from, 96, 113; abuse of, 102; abuse liability of, 94, 112–13; alcohol detoxification treatment, 107–9; avoidance of, in dementia, 61; —, in generalized anxiety disorder, 43; cross–tolerance with barbiturates of, 122; delirium due to, 53; delirium treatment, 58; detoxification from, 112–15; memory loss due to, 46; panic disorder treatment, 45–46; toxicology screen for, 103, 113; withdrawal potential of, 95
Beta blockers, 190, 191, 215, 224. See also Propranolol hydrochloride
Bipolar disorder: psychiatric referral for, 23; suicide in, 80; syndrome of, 15–16
Botulinum toxin, 224–25, 227
Botulism, 148–49
Brown-Séquard syndrome, 152, 161, 164
Bulbar signs, 146, 151–52
Buprenorphine hydrochloride, 110–11
Bupropion hydrochloride. See Antidepressants
Buspirone hydrochloride: for agitation in dementia, 61; for generalized anxiety disorder, 43
Butalbital, 103, 114, 192

Caffeine, 188–89, 192
"CAGE-B" questionnaire, 102–3
Calcium channel blockers, 180, 190, 191
Cancer: back pain due to, 174; and headaches, 180; major depression due to, 16; numbness due to, 159, 162; and suicide, 80; weakness due to, 146. See also Pheochromocytoma; Thymoma
Cannabis, 94, 96, 97
Carbamazepine: avoidance of, in alcohol detoxification, 109; —, in barbiturate and benzodiazepine detoxification, 114–15; in dementia, 61; for trigeminal neuralgia, 182
Carpal tunnel syndrome, 133, 142, 161, 167
Cataplexy, 204
Cauda equina syndrome, 159, 162, 169–70, 172, 174
Causalgia, 157
Cerebellum: functional anatomy of, 141; signs of damage to, 134
Cerebrovascular disease: dementia due to, 53; dizziness due to, 201, 202, 209–10; focal cognitive syndromes due to, 54; major depression due to, 16; neurologic referral for, 169–70; numbness due to, 162, 163; tremor due to, 226; weakness due to, 144, 154
Chlordiazepoxide hydrochloride: detoxification from, 113–14; for detoxification from alcohol, 107–8; toxicology screen for, 103
"Clasp knife" phenomenon, 139
Claudication, neurogenic, 176
Clonazepam: avoiding in detoxification from alcohol, 108–9; for detoxification from other benzodiazepines, 114; for panic disorder, 46; for tremor, 224, 228; toxicology screen for, 103; withdrawal potential of, 95

Clonidine, 112, 122
Cocaine: abstinence syndrome from, 96; abuse of, 102; abuse liability of, 94; antidepressants for withdrawal from, 109–10, 120; craving for, 99, 109; dependence and route of administration, 101–2; detoxification from, 109–10; panic attacks precipitated by, 39; and suicide, 109; toxicology screen for, 103; withdrawal causing major depression, 17, 109; withdrawal potential of, 95, 97
Cognitive-behavioral psychotherapy, 48
Cognitive testing: for dementia, 55–56; as part of neurologic examination, 135–36. See also Mini-Mental State Examination
Colchicine, 145
Compulsions, 39
Computed tomography. See Neuroimaging
Consciousness, disturbances of: and cerebral localization, 135; and midline reticular activating system, 134; evaluating on neurologic examination, 135. See also Delirium
Conversion disorder. See "Hysteria"
Coordination, 141–42
Corticosteroids: affective disorders due to, 16–17; delirium due to, 53; headache treatment, 180–81; tremor due to, 215; weakness due to, 145
Cranial nerves: examination of, 136–38, 142; false signs of damage to, 132
Creutzfeldt-Jakob disease, 58
Cushing syndrome, 16
Cyproheptadine, 190

Decongestants, 167, 186–87, 192
Delirium: causes of, 52–53; major depression distinguished from, 22; syndrome of, 51; treatment of, 58. See also Consciousness
Delusional disorder, somatic type, 72
Delusions: in Alzheimer disease, 60–61; asking about, 6, 21; defined, 6, 21; in delusional disorder, 72; in major depression, 14, 21, 54–55, 68, 72; in mania, 15; in schizophrenia, 72; treatment for, 58, 60–61
Dementia: assessment for, 54–56; caregivers for patients with, 60, 62–63; catastrophic reactions in, 60, 62; causes of, 53–54; course of, 56, 63; delusions in, 60–61; disordered behavior in, 60–61; evaluation explained to patients with, 56; language in, 5; major depression in, 60; in Parkinson disease, 222; specialist referral for, 55–57; support groups for, 62; syndrome of, 52; treatment of, 59–63
Demoralization: in caregivers for dementia patients, 62; as reaction to psychiatric referral, 74–75; in substance abuse relapse, 123, 124; and suicidal thoughts, 89
Dermatomyositis, 145
Desipramine hydrochloride: for cocaine abuse, 109; for panic disorder, 45
Diabetes mellitus: numbness due to, 159, 162; and small-fiber neuropathy, 133; weakness due to, 145
Diazepam: for detoxification, from alcohol, 107–8;

—, from other benzodiazepines, 113–14; toxicology screen for, 103; withdrawal potential of, 95
Dicyclomine hydrochloride, 112, 122
Diplopia, 137, 146, 151–52, 202
Disc, herniated: back pain due to, 172, 173, 174, 175; radiculopathy due to, 159; treatment of, 168, 174, 175–76
Disulfiram. See Alcohol
Divalproex sodium: for cluster headaches, 180; in dementia, 61
Dizziness: causes of, 197–207; differentiating features of, 198; examination of patient with, 209–10; experience of, 196, 197; as migraine manifestation, 185, 201, 202, 203; orthostatic, 202–3, 210; taking history of, 207–9; types of, 196–99
Dominant hemisphere lesions, 134
Donepezil hydrochloride, 59
Droperidol, 58
Dysarthria, 142, 151–52, 202, 226, 228
Dysesthesia, 157
Dysphagia, 151–52, 222
Dystonia, 227, 228

Electroencephalogram: in dementia, 55; in major depression, 22; in pseudoseizures, 212; in seizures, 201, 211–12; in sleep disorders, 204
Electromyography, 150, 153, 154, 176, 185–86, 228
Epilepsy. See Seizures
Ergotamines, 192
Extrapyramidal syndrome, 135

Fasciculations, 139, 146, 151
Fascioscapulohumeral dystrophy, 145
Fluoxetine hydrochloride: for major depression, 27, 28, 29, 32, 90; nortriptyline hydrochloride interaction, 31–32
Focal cognitive syndromes: progression to dementia, 63; treatment for, 63; types of, 52
Forgetfulness, normal, 63–64
Frontal lobes: dementias involving, 54; signs of damage to, 54, 134, 136

Ganglionopathy. See Peripheral nerve disorders
Gegenhalten, 139
Ginkgo biloba, 59, 60
Graphesthesia, 166
Guillain-Barré syndrome, 145, 148, 153–54, 159

Hallucinations: in Alzheimer disease, 60–61; asking about, 6; defined, 6; in delirium, 51; in Lewy body dementia, 53; in major depression, 14, 21; in mania, 15; in narcolepsy, 204; treatment for, 58, 61
Haloperidol, 58, 61
Headaches: caffeine withdrawal, 188–89; cluster, 180–81; and dizziness, 201, 202, 203; eliminating triggers of, 187–89; explaining mechanism to patients, 183–84, 194–95; idiopathic intracranial hypertension causing, 181; migraine, 162, 163, 182–94, 198, 203; myths about, 185–187; neu-

roimaging for, 179, 181, 186; neurologic referral for, 179–82; pathophysiology of, 182, 184–87; rebounding of, 182, 192–94; sinus, 183, 186–87; symptoms associated with, 180, 181, 185, 198, 203; temporal arteritis causing, 181; tension, 183, 185–86; treatment failures, 192–95; treatment of, 180–83, 187–95; types of, 179–85
Heroin. See Opioids
Herpes zoster, 159
Hippocampal sclerosis, idiopathic, 54
HMG-CoA reductase inhibitors, 145
Homunculus, 135, 162–63
Hopelessness: as reaction to psychiatric referral, 74; and suicide, 86
Human immunodeficiency virus: dementia due to, 54; and headaches, 180; major depression due to, 16; numbness due to, 159; substance abuse in patients with, 93; and suicide, 80
Huntington disease, 16, 80
Hydrocephalus, 54
Hydrocodone, 103, 175
Hydromorphone, 122
Hyperalgesia, 157
Hyperesthesia, 157
Hyperparathyroidism, 16, 54
Hyperpathia, 157, 159
Hyperthyroidism: anxiety disorders mimicked by, 40; false "cranial nerve signs" in, 132; sedative withdrawal mimicked by, 113; tremor from, 216, 228
Hyperventilation, 158, 206
Hypochondriasis. See Somatic symptoms
Hypoglycemia: anxiety disorders mimicked by, 40; dizziness due to, 203; seizures due to, 203; tremor from, 215
Hypomania. See Bipolar disorder
Hypoparathyroidism, 40
Hypothyroidism: dementia due to, 54, 55; major depression due to, 16, 22; and vague symptoms, 67
"Hysteria": as behavior, 69–70; as complaint of numbness, 164–65, 169; as conversion disorder, 70, 75–77; as pseudoseizures, 198, 205–6, 212; prevalence of, 71; as somatization disorder, 70–71, 75–77; treatment of, 75–77

Illusions: asking about, 6; defined, 6; in delirium, 51; treatment for, 58
Interferon-alpha, 16
International Tremor Foundation, 222
Isometheptene, 192

Jendrassik maneuver, 141

Lambert Eaton syndrome, 146
"Lead pipe" resistance, 139
Lewy bodies, 53–54
Lightheadedness, 197, 201
Lithium, 181, 216
Lorazepam: for delirium, 58; for detoxification from alcohol, 107–8; for panic disorder, 45

Magnetic resonance imaging. *See* Neuroimaging
Major depression: and anxiety disorders, 19, 38, 39; course of, 15, 18, 32–33; delirium distinguished from, 22; delusions in, 14, 21, 54–55, 68, 72; dementia due to, 54, 55; diagnosing, 17–22, 68; economic cost of, 14; epidemiology of, 13, 68; etiology of, 16–17; explaining to patients, 32–33; hallucinations in, 14, 21; laboratory studies for, 22; mental status examination for, 5, 19–21; in Parkinson disease, 16, 222; personality affected by, 4; psychiatric referral for, 23–24, 88; somatic symptoms in, 14, 17–18, 54–55, 66, 68, 72; substance abuse in, 17, 19, 115, 119; suicidal thoughts in, 20, 23, 85–86, 90; suicide in, 14, 80, 85, 90; syndrome of, 13–14; taking history of, 17–19; treatment of, 13, 14–15, 23, 24–33, 90, 109–10; in women who abuse alcohol, 115, 119
Malingering, 70, 150, 169, 205
Mania. *See* Bipolar disorder
Mental status examination: conducting, 5–11; for major depression, 5, 19–21; for obsessive-compulsive disorder, 39–40. *See also* Cognitive testing; Mini-Mental State Examination
Meralgia paresthetica, 161
Methadone: for heroin detoxification, 110–11; for opioid abuse relapse prevention, 120–21; toxicology screen for, 103
Methyldopa, 16
Methysergide, 180–81
Midazolam hydrochloride, 58
Migraines. *See* Headaches
Mini-Mental State Examination, 7–11, 136
Mitral valve prolapse, 41
Mononeuropathy. *See* Peripheral nerve disorders
Mood: assessment of, 5–6, 19–20; normal sadness as, 12
Morphine sulfate, 111–12
Motor neuron disease. *See* Amyotrophic lateral sclerosis
Motor system examination, 139–40, 149–52
Multiple sclerosis: barber's chair or Lhermitte's sign due to, 167; numbness due to, 162; and suicide, 80; tremor due to, 226; trigeminal neuralgia due to, 159; and vague symptoms, 67; weakness due to, 147
Muscular dystrophy, 145
Myasthenia gravis: bulbar signs due to, 151–52; fatigue in, 133; repetitive nerve stimulation testing for, 153–54; vague symptoms in, 67; weakness due to, 146, 150–51
Myelitis, transverse, 147, 148
Myelopathy: basic pattern of, 134, 150–51, 152; cervical, 147, 151, 168–69; neurologic referral for, 169–70
Myopathy: basic pattern of, 132, 150–51, 152; electromyography for, 153; false "cranial nerve signs" in, 132; types of, 145
Myositis, inclusion body, 145
Myotonic dystrophy, 145

Naltrexone hydrochloride: for alcohol craving, 117–18; for opioid abuse relapse prevention, 120, 121; stopping before surgery, 118, 123
Narcolepsy, 204
Narcotics Anonymous, 115–16, 119–20, 121
Nerve conduction tests, 145, 152–53, 154, 176
Nerve stimulation, repetitive, 153–54
Neuralgia: defined, 157; trigeminal, 159, 181–82
Neuroimaging: for back pain, 176; for dementia, 53, 55; for dizziness, 211; for headaches, 179, 181, 186; for major depression, 22; for seizures, 201
Neurologic evaluation: basic anatomic patterns shown by, 131–35, 150–52; physical examination in, 132, 135–43, 149–52, 166–67, 173, 209–10, 220–21; role of history in, 131, 147–48, 165–66, 172–73, 207–9, 216–20
Neurologist, referral to: for back pain, 172–77; for cranial nerve evaluation, 137; for headaches, 179–82; for numbness or tingling, 168–70; for tremor, 221, 224–26; for weakness, 140, 148–49, 150, 152, 154
Neuromuscular junction diseases: basic pattern of, 133, 150–51; repetitive nerve stimulation testing for, 153–54; weakness due to, 146. *See also* Myasthenia gravis
Neuropathy. *See* Peripheral nerve disorders
Neuropeptides, 184
Nicotine, 93, 94, 95, 96
Nondominant hemisphere lesions, 134
Nonsteroidal antiinflammatory drugs: for back pain, 174–75; for compressive neuropathies, 168; for headaches, 191, 192
Nortriptyline hydrochloride: for major depression, 25–26, 31, 32, 90; for migraine prevention, 190–91; for panic disorder, 45; selective serotonin reuptake inhibitor interaction with, 31–32; and suicide, 90
Numbness: causes of, 158–65; defined, 156–57; disabilities due to, 157; neurologic referral for, 168, 169–70. *See also* Peripheral nerve disorders; Sensation

Obsessions, 39
Obsessive-compulsive disorder. *See* Anxiety disorders
Olanzapine, 61
Opioids: abstinence syndrome from, 96; abuse of, group treatments, 115–16, 119–20; —, laboratory results suggesting, 102; —, methadone for, 120–21; —, naltrexone hydrochloride for, 120; —, signs suggesting, 102; abuse liability of, 94; back pain treatment, 175; craving for, 99, 122; and cross-tolerance to alcohol, 99; dependence on and route of administration, 101–2; detoxification from, 110–12; nonopioid medications for withdrawal from, 112, 122; postoperative use for opioid abusers, 122–23; and rebound headaches, 192, 193; toxicology screen for, 103, 112; withdrawal potential of, 95, 110
Osteophytes, 159, 177

Oxazepam: detoxification from, 113–14; for detoxification from alcohol, 107–8; for panic disorder, 45
Oxycodone hydrochloride: for back pain, 175; detoxification from, 111; for detoxification from other opioids, 111–12

Panic disorder. *See* Anxiety disorders
Paresthesia: in benzodiazepine withdrawal, 113; causes of, 158–62, 167, 185; defined, 156–57; experience of, 157; in panic disorder, 38. *See also* Peripheral nerve disorders; Sensation
Parietal lobe: and discriminative sensory modalities, 166; signs of damage to, 135–36, 137, 163
Parkinson disease: delirium caused by treatments for, 53; dementia due to, 54; and Lewy body dementia, 53; major depression due to, 16. *See also* Tremor
Peripheral nerve disorders: axonal, 145–46, 153; basic patterns of, 133, 145–46, 151–52, 156–65; compressive, 159, 162, 168–70; dementia with, 55; demyelinating, 145–46, 153; electromyography for, 153; ganglionopathy, 162; large-fiber, 133–34, 142, 158–59, 164, 166; mononeuropathy, 158–59, 168; mononeuropathy multiplex, 158–60, 162; nerve conduction testing for, 152–53; neurologic referral for, 169–70; numbness or tingling due to, 157–62; plexopathy, 150, 159, 162; radiculopathy, 150, 159, 162, 168–69, 173, 176–77, 187; small-fiber, 133–34, 142, 158–59, 164, 166; stocking-glove sensory loss in, 145, 152, 158, 160; symmetric, 158–59; treatment of, 167–69; weakness due to, 145–46. *See also* Guillain-Barré syndrome
Paroxetine hydrochloride: for generalized anxiety disorder, 44; for major depression, 27–29, 90; nortriptyline hydrochloride interaction, 31–32; for panic disorder, 45
Personality: "addictive," 100; change as sign of prefrontal dysfunction, 54, 136; inquiring about, 4; and vulnerability to adjustment disorder with depressed mood, 12
Phenobarbital: for detoxification from other barbiturates, 114; as primidone metabolite, 223; toxicology screen for, 103
Phenytoin: avoiding in detoxification, from alcohol, 109, 117; —, from barbiturates and benzodiazepines, 114–15; for trigeminal neuralgia, 182
Pheochromocytoma: mimicking anxiety disorders, 40, 41; tremor from, 215
Pick disease, 54
Plexopathy. *See* Peripheral nerve disorders
Polymyalgia rheumatica, 181
Polymyositis, 132, 145
Posterior fossa lesions, basic pattern of, 134, 163, 226
Posttraumatic stress disorder, 36, 47
Presyncope. *See* Syncope
PRIME-MD screening questionnaire, 41
Primidone, 223–24
Pronator drift, 140
Propranolol hydrochloride: avoiding in detoxification, from alcohol, 109; —, from barbiturates and

benzodiazepines, 114–15; for essential tremor, 223–24; major depression due to, 16; for migraine prophylaxis, 190
Pseudotumor cerebri, 181
Psychiatric history: obtaining, 3–4; screening approach to, 41–42
Psychiatrist, referral to: for anxiety disorders, 47–48; for caregivers of patients with dementia, 62–63; for dementia, 56–57; for major depression, 23–24, 88; preparing patients for, 72–76; for substance use disorders, 88, 104, 114–16, 121; for suicidal thoughts, 87–89; for unexplained somatic symptoms, 72–77
Psychoactive substances: abstinence syndromes from, 96; abuse of, 97; abuse liability of, 94–95, 97; characteristics of, 93–97; craving for, 99; cross-tolerance among, 98–99; dependence on, 97–100; detoxification from, 105–15; diagnosing use of, 102–3; discussing use with patients, 103–5; dizziness due to, 198, 203–4; prevalence of use, 93; risk factors for, 100–101; taking usage history, 101; tolerance to, 95, 98–99; toxicology screen for, 103; tremor in withdrawal from, 215; withdrawal potential of, 95, 97
Psychomotor retardation, 20
Ptosis, 137, 146, 151–52, 180

Radiculopathy. *See* Peripheral nerve disorders
Reaction, catastrophic, 60, 62
Reflexes, examination of, 140–41
Renal failure: delirium due to, 52; dementia due to, 54; and suicide, 80; weakness due to, 145
Reserpine, 16
Riluzole, 147
Risperidone, 58, 61

Schizophrenia, 72, 80
Sciatica, 175–76
Secobarbital. *See* Barbiturates
Seizures, epileptic: absence, 200–201, 211; alcohol withdrawal, 109; complex partial, 198, 200–201, 204; dizziness due to, 198–201; focal, 200, 211–12; myoclonic, 201, 211; numbness due to, 163; pseudoseizures, 198, 205–6, 212; simple partial, 199–200; tonic-clonic, 198–203, 205–6, 209, 211
Selective serotonin reuptake inhibitors. *See* Antidepressants
Selegiline hydrochloride, 59
Self-attitude, 14, 15, 20, 21
Sensation, examination of, 142–43, 152, 160–61, 164–67
Sertraline hydrochloride: for generalized anxiety disorder, 44; nortriptyline hydrochloride interaction, 31–32; for major depression, 27–29, 90; for panic disorder, 45
Sexual drive: selective serotonin reuptake inhibitors affecting, 27–29; in major depression, 17–18; in mania, 15
Shoulder, painful, 150

Sign: barber's chair, 167; bulbar, 146, 151–52; Lhermitte's, 167–68; Phalen's, 161, 167; Tinel's, 161, 167

Sjögren syndrome, 159, 162

Sleep, disordered: after detoxification from alcohol, 116; in generalized anxiety disorder, 37; in major depression, 17; narcolepsy causing, 204; night terrors causing, 204; periodic limb movements causing, 204; treatment in dementia, 61

Social phobia. *See* Anxiety disorders

Somatic symptoms: in anxiety disorders, 36–39, 66, 68–69; in delusional disorder, 72; epidemiology of, 66, 71; in "hysteria," 69–71, 75–76; in major depression, 14, 17–18, 66, 68; psychiatric referral for, 72–77; in schizophrenia, 72; treatment of psychiatric disorders underlying, 75–76

Somatization disorder. *See* "Hysteria"

Spinal cord, signs of partial damage to, 163–64. *See also* Myelopathy; Stenosis

"Spinal shock," 134, 141

Spondylosis, lumbar, 176–77

Stenosis: cervical, 134, 145, 147, 148, 150–51, 168–69; lumbar, 176

Stereognosis, 166

Stimulation, deep brain, 225

Stokes-Adams attacks, 202

Subdural hematoma, 54

Substance abuse: denial of, 104; dependency syndrome in, 98–100; diagnosing, 102–3; discussing with patients, 103–5; family intervention for, 104; group treatments for, 115–16, 118–20; hypnotics, opioids, and sedatives in, 121–23; laboratory tests for, 102–3; motivation for treatment of, 125–26; and psychiatric comorbidity, 17, 19, 115, 119; recovery from, 116, 123–24; regarding as disease, 104–5; relapse prevention, 115–23; relapse treatment, 123–24; risk factors for, 100–101; social consequences of, 98, 101; specialist referral for, 88, 104, 114–16, 121; and suicide, 80, 85, 109

Suicidal thoughts: asking about, 4, 6, 81–86, 91; interventions for, 86–91; involuntary hospitalization for, 23, 88; in major depression, 19, 20, 23, 85–86, 90; and medical illness, 80–81, 89; psychiatric referral for, 23–24, 87–89

Suicide: epidemiology of, 79–81, 85; family history of, 3, 18; and hopelessness, 86; in major depression, 14, 90; in panic disorder, 49; medical disorders associated with, 80–81; most common means of, 79; psychiatric disorders associated with, 80; risk for, 83–86, 90; and substance abuse, 80, 85, 109

Sumatriptan, 180, 191, 192

Syncope, 198, 200, 202–3, 208, 209

Syndrome. *See specific syndrome*

Syphilis, 54

Syringomyelia, 161, 164

Systemic lupus erythematosus, 67, 80

Tacrine hydrochloride, 59

Temporomandibular joint dysfunction, 187

Test: Rinne, 138; Romberg, 142; "swinging flashlight," 136; Weber, 138

Thalamic pain, 163

Thalamotomy, stereotactic, 225

Theophylline, 216

Thiothixene, 61

Thoracic outlet syndrome, 161

Thymoma, 146

Tingling. *See* Paresthesia

Tinnitus, 185, 197, 202

Traction, cervical, 169

Transient ischemic attack. *See* Cerebrovascular disease

Trazodone hydrochloride, 61, 116, 122

Tremor: causes of, 214–16; cerebellar, 215, 226; characterization of, 214–15; dystonic, 227; enhanced physiologic, 214–16; essential, 214–25; intention, 215, 226; kinetic, 215–16, 226, 228; in Parkinson disease, 214–22, 225; primary orthostatic, 227–28; primary writing, 227; senile, 219; specialist referral for, 221, 224–26, 229; support group for, 222; treatment of, 222–25; Wilson disease causing, 228–29

Triazolam, 103, 112, 114

Tricyclics. *See* Antidepressants; Desipramine hydrochloride; Nortriptyline hydrochloride

Valproic acid, 216

Venlafaxine hydrochloride. *See* Antidepressants

Vertigo, 197, 201, 202

Vestibular disease, 198, 202

Vitamin E, 59, 60

Weakness: electrodiagnostic tests for, 152–54; "giveway," 150; neurologic disorders causing, 144–47; neurologic referral for, 150, 154; nonneurologic disorders causing, 149–50; patterns of, 144–45, 148–52; physical examination for, 139–40, 149–52; taking history of, 147–49. *See also* Myelopathy; Myopathy; Neuromuscular junction diseases; Peripheral nerve disorders

William's flexion exercises, 176

Wilson disease, 216, 228–29

Writer's cramp, 227